AWAKENING DESIRE: MASTERING THE NUANCES OF FOREPLAY FOR WOMEN

A Guide to Deepening Intimacy and Enhancing Pleasure"

GRISELDA W. GRIMALDO

Table of Contents

Copyright

Griselda W. Grimaldo's copyright © 2024

Disclaimer

Awakening Desire: Mastering the Nuances of Foreplay in Women is a book that provides material solely for educational and informative reasons. It is not meant to replace professional medical advice, diagnosis, or treatment. The information in this book should not be construed as therapeutic or medical advice because the author and publisher are not trained counselors, sex therapists, or medical experts.

Professional Advice

Readers seeking individualized guidance and assistance are advised to speak with a licensed healthcare professional or sex therapist. It's crucial to get expert help if you have any health difficulties, sexual dysfunction, or relationship problems.

Individual Differences

Sexuality is a highly personal and intricate component of human existence, and it may elicit a broad range of individual experiences, preferences, and reactions. Readers are advised to respect each other's comfort zones and boundaries and speak honestly with their partners, as not everyone will find success with the methods and ideas presented in this book.

Safety and Consent

This book's material highlights how crucial respect, communication, and mutual consent are to any sexual activity. It is essential to ensure that partners always feel safe and at ease and that all interactions are consensual. Any activities that are uncomfortable or upsetting should be discontinued immediately, and any issues should be discussed in an open forum.

Accountability

The author or publisher is not responsible for any adverse effects or repercussions arising from the use or abuse of the material included in this book. Readers should exercise caution when utilizing the offered strategies and recommendations, as they are ultimately accountable for their own choices and actions.

Age Appropriateness

This book is meant for adult readers only and includes explicit content. Those under the age of eighteen should not use it. Any information about sexuality should be age-appropriate and appropriate for younger readers; therefore, parents and guardians should ensure this.

By reading this book, you accept the disclaimer and its conditions and realize how important it is to get expert help for any problems relating to your personal health or relationships.

Preface

Welcome, Reader. "Awakening Desire: Mastering the Nuances of Foreplay for Women" gives me great pleasure to invite you to embark on this journey of inquiry into the subtleties of pleasure, proximity, and longing. This book is a labor of love, the product of a great need to acknowledge and respect the range of experiences connected to sexuality that women have. On these pages, you will find a wealth of knowledge, viewpoints, and practical advice that will help you to become closer to your body, goals, and limits.

Foreplay is crucial for reaching the highest level of sexual pleasure and closeness, even if it is sometimes overlooked or underrated. Using touch, communication, and sensory augmentation, we may excite desire, fire passion, and create close bonds with our partners.

As you start your journey, I implore you to approach these teachings with an open mind and a curious attitude. Take advantage of the opportunity to challenge preconceptions, investigate fresh viewpoints, and determine what makes your close relationships happy and fulfilling.

Remember that your path of sexual discovery is unique to you and that no two people feel desire or pleasure in the same way. Trust your gut sense, respect your limits, and embrace the complete spectrum of your needs guilt-free.

Above all, I hope this book will be a source of validation, inspiration, and empowerment for women everywhere attempting to grasp the complexities of foreplay and ignite their desire. With curiosity, self-assurance, and an uncompromising commitment to your happiness and fulfillment, I hope it gives you the bravery to embrace your sexuality.

Yours Sincerely

Best wishes.

Griselda W. Grimaldo

AN ACCOUNT OF AWAKENING LONGING

Lena and Mark were now together eight years after they started dating. From the wild whirl of undergraduate enthusiasm, their partnership had evolved into a strong alliance defined by respect for one another, shared goals, and great devotion. Their once-passionate connection started to wane, though, as they grew used to the routines of adult life—which entailed balancing work, housekeeping, and occasionally family member chores.

Lena first noticed the change late in the evening on a crisp autumn night. Mark and she were drinking hot chocolate while seated on their terrace, covered in blankets. As was typical, the discussion veered from business and chores to more introspective themes. Lena decided to raise the subject since she missed their passionate, spontaneous relationship. "Recall our first trip to the mountains together?" With a melancholic expression, she enquired.

Mark nodded, his eyes sparkling. Naturally, I do. After straying on that hiking path, we saw a fantastic waterfall. That one was one of the best weekends we have ever had.

Lena sighed, but her smile lost some brightness. " There used to be a lot of spark and excitement between us. I forget that occasionally. Mark held out his hand to grab hers. I miss it as well, Lena. One's life has gotten somewhat busy. That does not imply that we cannot fan that flame again. That evening's conversation began a road for them—a conscious decision to rediscover their intimacy and go farther into their marriage. They decided to start with a simple but essential commitment: schedule time to rediscover one another as lovers instead of as friends.

"Awakening Desire" invites you to embrace the personal journey open-minded and emotionally accessible. Foreplay is not only a precursor for sex; it is a necessary component of a loving and fulfilling marriage. Learning the nuances of foreplay will help you build your link with your partner, enhance your sexual experiences, and establish a relationship full of love and pleasure.

This book is your road map for that journey; it offers techniques, ideas, and helpful advice to overcome the obstacles of foreplay effectively. This is a call to explore the depths of intimacy, open, honest communication, and create a close relationship with the person you love. As you strive for a more passionate and fulfilling relationship, I hope it proves to be a helpful tool for you.

NOBODY HAS A PHYSIQUE OR PASSION LIKE A WOMAN. LISTEN CAREFULLY AND WATCH HER EMOTIONS DURING PRIVATE MOMENTS TO LEARN WHAT EXCITES HER MOST.

CHAPTER 1

THE ESSENTIAL ROLE OF FOREPLAY

Intimacy is a sacred art form, and foreplay is frequently considered the prelude to this symphony. An art form that goes beyond physical touch to cover the depths of emotional and psychological connection, it is a delicate dance of anticipation, exploration, and desire. The complex web of sexual intimacy begins with foreplay, which is especially important for women since it lays the groundwork for more meaningful connections.

At its core, foreplay is not just about getting the body ready for sexual activity but also about getting the mind and spirit prepared for the journey of intimacy. For women, foreplay is a crucial aspect of arousal, desire, and bonding with their partners emotionally. This is a chance to learn, grow, be vulnerable, and establish trust.

One of the primary purposes of foreplay in women is to bridge the gap between their inner and outer worlds of desire. Modern women may find it challenging to fully immerse themselves in the here and now due to our fast-paced society's abundance of distractions and responsibilities. They can slow down, disconnect from the stresses of daily life, and rediscover their connection to their bodies and desires through foreplay.

During foreplay, ladies can let their innate sensuality and erotica shine through intimate touches and movements.

The borders separating desire and self-control, as well as between pain and pleasure, are being blurred during this era of experimentation and discovery. Women can learn to enjoy their sexuality without shame or inhibition by exploring their bodies, finding new erogenous zones, and perfecting the art of foreplay.

For women, emotional connection is also another critical component of foreplay. Women's sexual arousal is directly tied to their emotional condition, in contrast to men, who usually experience more instantaneous and physical excitement. Women can entirely yield to the experience of intimacy when they feel safe, trusted, and emotionally bonded to their partner. Couples can develop their emotional connection, express their love and affection through touch, and freely explore their desires and fantasies during foreplay. It is a phase of openness and honesty when couples can remove their boundaries and connect on a soul-deep level. Couples can create a deeper degree of closeness and understanding via the art of foreplay, setting the groundwork for a satisfying and gratifying sexual relationship.

 Moreover, foreplay plays a critical function in bridging the emotional and physical components of sexual intimacy. It's a period of change when a desire's first spark turns into a fierce flame. Couples can create anticipation and excitement, heighten arousal, and strengthen their bond by touching sensually, making personal motions, and whispering words of love to one another. Foreplay is vital for women, in particular, to reach the highest potential levels of arousal and pleasure. Women's arousal patterns tend to be more nuanced and changeable than men's, who frequently demonstrate more linear and predictable sexual reactions. To fully awaken the body to the delights of intimacy, one must dedicate time, patience, and care.

Women who manage foreplay can gradually build their degree of arousal, with feelings increasing stronger as time goes on. It facilitates the development of a more profound sense of pleasure and satisfaction and the research of various erogenous zones and fresh sensations. Couples can create a more pleasurable and rewarding sexual session for both parties by dedicating time and energy to foreplay.

Furthermore, foreplay is an efficient approach for getting past everyday impediments to sexual intimacy, like tension, weariness, and distraction. It can be challenging for couples in today's bustling world to find time for intimacy between the constraints of employment, family, and other commitments. During foreplay, couples can settle down, re-establish their connection, and give their relationship priority.

Couples can build intimacy and connection that goes beyond the physical through sensual touch, intense conversation, and shared experiences. At this season of regeneration and refreshment, couples can escape the cares of everyday life and indulge in the delights of intimacy. By prioritizing foreplay in their relationship, couples can improve communication, fortify their tie, and develop a deeper connection.

In conclusion, it is hard to exaggerate the value of foreplay in women. It is the doorway to pleasure, the link between intimate physical and emotional interactions, and the cornerstone of more meaningful partnerships. By mastering the art of foreplay, women can excite their libido, improve their bond with their partners, and enjoy a great feeling of pleasure and fulfillment. It's a period of discovery, transparency, and sincerity—a heavenly spot where want and love meet.

On their journey to recover the art of foreplay, Lena and Mark engaged in research and learning. To get a knowledge of the psychology and science underlying sexual desire, they started by reading books and articles on the issue. They discovered that arousal is highly influenced by foreplay, especially in women, who usually need a mix of physical and emotional cues to trigger a sexual response.

How to Use This Guide

"Awakening Desire" is designed to walk you through the many parts of foreplay, covering everything from the psychological and biological bases to the practical strategies and emotional factors. Every chapter builds on the one before it, delivering a complete plan for grasping and improving foreplay.

Regardless of how long you have been dating or how recently you started dating, this book provides incisive analysis and valuable suggestions that you can modify to your personal relationship's particulars. It fosters self- and mutual exploration, creating the openness and curiosity essential for a fulfilling and dynamic love life.

CHAPTER 2

THE SIGNS OF AROUSAL UNDERSTANDING: UNDERSTANDING FEMALE PHYSIOLOGY

"Awakening Desire" is a comprehensive guide that will walk you through all aspects of foreplay, from its biological and psychological foundation to its practical strategies and emotional components. Each chapter expands upon the previous one, providing a thorough approach to understanding and enhancing foreplay. No matter how long you've been dating or how recently you started dating, this book offers helpful advice and intelligent analysis that you can tailor to the specifics of your relationship. It fosters self- and mutual exploration, cultivating an openness and curiosity essential for a happy and dynamic love life.

Like many other couples, Lena and Mark set out to reclaim the closeness and passion that had once characterized their union. They found themselves learning more about the subtleties of foreplay and the mysteries of female arousal. Lena thought that knowing the physics of arousal was enlightening and gave her a chance to re-establish a deep connection with her body and wants. Lena and Mark learned that female arousal is a complicated, nuanced process that is influenced by a wide range of factors as they set out on their quest. Factors, including hormone changes, emotional states, and sensory cues, shaped Lena's perception of arousal and desire.

Hormonal Dynamics: The Function of Estrogen and Testosterone

The hormones testosterone and estrogen, which both have specific roles in controlling sexual function, are at the core of female arousal. Estrogen, also known as the "female hormone," is in charge of preserving vaginal lubrication, improving touch sensitivity, and fostering general sexual health. Lena discovered that variations in her estrogen levels throughout her menstrual cycle can significantly affect her receptivity to sexual stimuli. Traditionally linked to masculine sexuality, testosterone is essential for female pleasure as well. Testosterone, which is produced in the adrenal glands and ovaries, has a role in arousal, libido, and general sexual satisfaction. Lena found that her testosterone levels affected her receptivity and desire, underscoring the significance of hormonal balance in sexual wellness.

The Power of Oxytocin: Creating Emotional Connection

While studying arousal, Lena and Mark also learned about the powerful impact of the "love hormone" oxytocin on female sexual response. Oxytocin, which is released during intimate and bonding situations, promotes emotions of emotional closeness, trust, and connection. Lena discovered that her experience of pleasure was more prosperous and more satisfying when she felt loved, respected, and emotionally linked to Mark. Lena and Mark found the importance of emotional connection during intimate times and how it dramatically affects Lena's level of arousal and enjoyment. They developed an intimacy that prepared the way for more significant and in-depth interactions by showing affection, talking, and sharing experiences.

Dopamine and Pleasure: Enhancing Sensations and Desire

Dopamine, sometimes known as the "pleasure hormone," is essential for female arousal. Dopamine is a neurotransmitter that is released in reaction to pleasurable stimuli. It increases feelings of pleasure and desire by producing exhilaration and contentment. Lena found that her passion for Mark increased when she experienced intimacy and connection, which caused a dopamine release. Lena and Mark played with various sensory stimuli as they investigated the function of dopamine in arousal, trying to find ways to increase Lena's enjoyment and contentment. They found that dopamine shaped Lena's perception of arousal in a variety of ways, from sensual contact to erotic imagery, providing new opportunities for communication and exploration.

The Psychological Triggers of Desire

Although hormones are essential in controlling arousal, Lena and Mark also found that psychological factors significantly impact how desire feels. Lena's perception and reaction to sexual stimuli are shaped by her emotions, ideas, memories, and past experiences, which collectively influence her sensation of desire and pleasure. The Basis of Desire: Emotional Bonding Lena believed that emotional closeness was an essential step before sexual desire. She felt safe and trusted with Mark because she felt loved, respected, and emotionally linked to him, which let her enjoy the feeling of intimacy to the fullest. Lena discovered that as their emotional connection grew, so did her desire for Mark, which increased her arousal and gave her a sense of thrill and anticipation.

Fantasy and Imagination: Exploring Desires and Fantasies

When it comes to arousal, the mind is an incredibly potent instrument that may evoke vivid fantasies and spark the imagination. Lena found that imagination gave her a safe, accepting environment in which to explore her fantasies and needs. Lena found new ways to increase her excitement and strengthen her bond with Mark through erotic books, vivid imagery, and creative storytelling.

Sensory Stimulation: Engaging the Senses

Lena's arousal is greatly influenced by her senses; aroma, taste, touch, sound, and sight all contribute to her total sensory perception. Lena and Mark found that by using several senses at once, they could enhance the inclusion and enjoyment of the experience, raising Lena's arousal and strengthening her bond with Mark.

Context and Environment: Creating the Perfect Atmosphere

Lena's perception of arousal can be significantly influenced by the environment in which sexual activity takes place; seclusion, comfort, and ambiance are a few examples of the elements that shape the mood and atmosphere. Lena and Mark discovered that establishing an intimate space, such as a warm bedroom with calming music and lighting, could raise Lena's arousal and encourage relaxation, strengthening their bond and sense of fulfillment.

Past Experiences: Overcoming Barriers to Desire
Ultimately, Lena and Mark learned that Lena's perception of and reaction to sexual stimuli can be influenced by her past experiences, both good and bad. Positive experiences can increase feelings of safety and trust, whereas traumatic ones—like sexual assault or abuse—can create barriers to arousal and closeness. Lena and Mark were able to work on removing obstacles to arousal and fostering a more satisfying sexual relationship by admitting and dealing with their past traumas.

The complex dynamics behind female desire can be fascinatingly glimpsed through the lens of arousal science. All factors, from hormone dynamics to psychological triggers, determine how Lena experiences arousal and fulfillment. Lena and Mark were able to develop a more pleasant and fulfilling sexual relationship by improving Lena's arousal and strengthening their connection via a better knowledge of the interaction between physiological and psychological elements. They opened the door to greater intimacy and connection by discovering the mysteries of pleasure through investigation, dialogue, and understanding.

CREATE A SENSE OF ANTICIPATION TO HEIGHTEN THE THRILL. ONE WAY TO HEIGHTEN AROUSAL AND STRENGTHEN THE CONNECTION IS WITH GENTLE TEASING AND PATIENT DEVELOPMENT.

CHAPTER 3

BUILDING EMOTIONAL INTIMACY

Emotional intimacy is the cornerstone of stronger partnerships in the context of human connection. In this holy space, vulnerability is accepted, trust is established, and connection deepens. Developing emotional closeness is essential for couples looking to fortify their relationship because it makes them feel closer, more sympathetic, and more supportive of one another.

Connection, Vulnerability, and Trust

Trust is the cornerstone of emotional intimacy; it is a deep belief in the reliability, integrity, and goodness of one's partner. Trust is the foundation of healthy relationships because it makes individuals feel secure and at ease, which motivates them to be honest and open with one another. Regarding partnerships that aim for emotional intimacy, trust is the foundation that helps deeper attachments grow.

Vulnerability is another essential component of emotional connection. It is having the courage to share one's innermost feelings, concerns, and ideas with someone without fear of rejection or condemnation. Vulnerability requires bravery and honesty because it allows one to be seen and welcomed for who they are. The embrace of vulnerability is the first step toward genuine connection, a deep understanding, acceptance, and empathy that transcends the superficial levels of interpersonal communication. Encouraging a sense of openness and vulnerability is essential for couples looking to get closer emotionally. It involves creating a safe and supportive environment where both partners feel comfortable speaking openly and honestly. Kindness, empathy, and compassion foster a sense of trust and vulnerability in a marriage, which lays the groundwork for a deeper emotional connection.

Breaking Through Emotional Obstacles
Though emotional closeness has many advantages, many couples encounter roadblocks, including fears, uncertainties, and traumatic experiences that keep them from forging a solid link. These emotional roadblocks can manifest in various ways, including difficulty expressing feelings, a fear of rejection, or a reluctance to trust others. Yet if they have the required tolerance, understanding, and encouragement from one another, couples may overcome these challenges and become closer and more connected. The fear of vulnerability is a common emotional barrier to intimacy. Many believe being honest with others would leave them exposed and helpless and that vulnerability equates to weakness. As a result, individuals would keep their lovers at a distance to shield them from hurt or rejection.

In overcoming this challenge, couples must create a safe, supportive space where vulnerability is acknowledged and cherished. They may do this by using active listening, empathy, and validation techniques to convey to their partners that their thoughts and emotions are respected and appreciated. By being vulnerable, couples may foster an environment where both parties feel comfortable sharing and being open.

A common emotional barrier to intimacy is fear of rejection. Numerous individuals harbor a profound apprehension of experiencing rejection once more due to earlier rejections in friendships, relationships, or other spheres of life. This anxiety might manifest as a reluctance to trust others, a fear of intimacy, or a tendency to push people away before they get too close. Couples must practice understanding, compassion, and tolerance to overcome this barrier. They need to accept that fear of rejection is a familiar human feeling that arises from concerns and unpleasant experiences from the past. They should also provide their partner's unconditional love and support while they work through these fears. By acting consistently, reliably, and with respect, couples may gradually build trust and create a sense of safety that allows both partners to open up and connect more intimately with one another.

In addition to fear of rejection and vulnerability, fears and prior traumas can create emotional barriers to closeness. These traumas, which might have their roots in early life experiences, past relationships, or other situations, can leave victims feeling wounded, suspicious, and unwilling to trust others. But with a loving and supportive partner, people may overcome their traumas and forge more incredible bonds of emotional intimacy.

Couples must practice active listening, empathy, and patience to overcome these challenges. They must create a warm, inviting environment where both partners feel free to share their thoughts and feelings without fear of rejection or condemnation. Through honest and open communication, couples may work together to heal past wounds, build trust, and create a stronger, more durable connection.

Emotional intimacy is a process that takes time to develop and involves trust, vulnerability, and connection. To enhance emotional closeness, a couple must be understanding, patient, and encouraging of one another. By creating a safe, supportive environment where both partners feel comfortable sharing and being vulnerable with one another, couples may overcome emotional barriers and forge a deeper, more meaningful connection. Emotional intimacy fosters the development of true love and understanding; these connections are enduring and transcend surface-level affection.

CHAPTER 4

TOUCH AND SENSATION: A JOURNEY OF INTIMATE EXPLORATION

Touch is the language of desire in the intricate dance of human closeness. It is a powerful tool for raising arousal, reinforcing emotional bonds, and fostering a sense of intimacy between partners. Touch can generate pleasure, stimulate the senses, and create personal moments. It may take many different forms, from the gentle caress of a lover's hand to a passionate kiss.

Overview of Touch: The Love Language

Touch is one of the most fundamental forms of communication and may convey a wide range of emotions, such as passion, desire, and love. From the time of our birth, touch has a significant influence on our development, shaping both our sense of ourselves and how the outside world seems to us. In romantic relationships, touch takes on a greater significance to express closeness, affection, and desire. Through touch, couples may express their love for one another, fortify their emotional connection, and relish the profound pleasure of physical intimacy.

Finding Erogenous Zones: Charting the Course for Happiness

The areas of the body that can produce pleasurable feelings and are exceptionally responsive to touch are erogenous zones. From the lips to the fingers, countless erogenous zones all over the body are just waiting to be discovered and investigated. Being a master of touch requires you to identify and activate these erogenous zones. Each person's body is unique, with sensitive areas that respond to touch differently. Probing their partner's body with interest and care could help people discover these hidden joys and create moments of intense closeness and connection.

Typical erogenous zones consist of:

1. The lips are among the body's most sensitive parts, and they can experience a wide range of feelings, from mild kisses to powerful bites. Gently petting, kissing, and nibbling the lips can stimulate feelings of desire and anticipation that enhance the pleasure of intimate partnerships.

2. The neck is another susceptible area commonly ignored in intimate partnerships. Tender kisses, nibbles, and caresses along the neck can foster intimate sentiments of closeness and connection between partners.

3. The ear is a susceptible part of the body that may be pleasurable when lightly touched, spoken, or kissed. Whispering sweet nothings, following the contours of the ear with the fingertips, and stimulating the sensation of closeness and earlobe play may all enhance the pleasure of intimate meetings.

4. The Nipples: Despite their extraordinary sensitivity to touch, many people find considerable pleasure in their nipples. Caressing, kissing, and nibbling the nipples softly can promote intimacy, desire, and delightful feelings.

5. The Inner Thighs: The inner thighs are a susceptible area of the body that is frequently ignored in intimate partnerships. Caresses, kisses, and nibbles down the inner thighs can produce a sense of anticipation and desire that will make intimate meetings more enjoyable.

6. Genitalia: The body's most sensitive erogenous zone, the genitalia can feel highly pleasurable touches, kisses, and caresses. Intimate and very satisfying moments can result from lovers probing these locations with care and attention. By thoughtfully and attentively exploring these erogenous zones, people can find new pleasures and create personal moments with their partners.

Developing Your Touch Skills: The Art of Sensual Investigation

The skill of touch must be mastered if one is to produce moments of intense pleasure and connection during intimate interactions. How touch is applied—from gentle caresses to forceful strokes—can have a significant impact on the amount of pleasure and arousal experienced. Developing touch approaches requires two essential skills: being in the moment and observing your partner's emotions. You may infer what makes them happy by paying attention to their vocalizations, body language, and verbal cues.

Among the techniques for developing touch proficiency are:

1. Gentle Caresses: Gentle caresses use delicate, featherlike touches to stimulate the skin and produce a sense of anticipation and excitement. Gently tracing patterns with the fingertips, feathering kisses all over the body, and sliding fingertips down the skin may all generate moments of intense pleasure and connection between lovers.

2. Firm Strokes: Firm strokes involve slightly more pressure to stimulate the skin and provide deep relaxation and pleasure. Using the palms of your hands or the pads of your fingers softly kneaded into the skin, you may feel intense pleasure and relaxation as you work on your muscles and skin.

3. Sensual Massage: This kind of massage stimulates the senses and creates deep relaxation using various methods. Lovers who use massage oils or lotions, long, flowing strokes, gentle kneading, and compression methods can feel intense pleasure and intimacy.

4. Teasing and Anticipation: This technique uses soft touches, kisses, and caresses to arouse and induce a sense of anticipation. By softly tracing the fingertips over the skin, gently kissing the lips, and lightly sliding the tongue down the body, one may produce moments of intense pleasure and excitement.

5. Exploration and Experimentation: This strategy involves trying several methods to identify what both spouses find amusing and pleasant. Learning these touch and exploration techniques can generate intensely pleasurable and connecting moments in intimate

experiences, strengthening their emotional attachment and increasing their sense of intimacy with their partners. Couples can create moments of tremendous pleasure and connection by experimenting with different techniques, exploring new erogenous zones, and trying different touches.

Breaking Through Emotional Obstacles: The Way to Closeness

Emotional barriers often prevent people from experiencing the complete intimacy of intimate encounters and from letting go, obstructing the joy and connection that can be felt. These challenges can manifest in a variety of ways, including anxiety, a fear of showing weakness, and difficulties putting your faith in others. They may also be the outcome of past worries, fears, and traumas. These emotional barriers must be crossed for intimate interactions to yield moments of deep pleasure and connection. It requires being willing to take on these challenges head-on, acknowledge and accept the underlying emotions, and set healing and advancement as the ultimate objectives.

Among the strategies for overcoming emotional barriers are:
1. Open and Honest Communication: If people are not upfront and honest with one another, they will not be able to express their worries, fears, or desires in a safe and supportive setting without fear of judgment or rejection. By promoting honest and open conversation, couples may

create a climate of trust and understanding that is a foundation for fortifying their emotional link and overcoming emotional barriers to intimacy.

2. Building Trust: Building trust is necessary to get beyond emotional barriers to intimacy. Trust requires being open and vulnerable, exposing one's deepest fears and weaknesses, and relying on others for consolation and support. People may cultivate trust and a sense of safety and security by acting honorably, dependably, and consistently in their relationships.

3. Developing Self-Compassion: Self-compassion means being accepting, tolerant, and gracious toward oneself, especially when one is feeling weak and self-conscious. By cultivating self-compassion, people may learn to affirm their emotions, accept and appreciate their flaws, and forgive themselves for past sins.

4. Seeking Expert Help: Speaking with a Licensed Counselor or Therapist: Sometimes, their assistance is necessary to overcome emotional barriers to closeness. Therapy may help people cope with underlying emotional issues, heal from past traumas, and form more positive thinking and behavior patterns by giving them the necessary tools, support, and guidance.

5. Self-Exploration: Self-exploration comprises thinking back on one's preferences, boundaries, and wants and openly and honestly addressing them with one's partner. By examining their own goals and desires, people may create opportunities for a better understanding of themselves and their relationship and for stronger emotional connection and intimacy. By intentionally working to get beyond these emotional obstacles and

fostering moments of deep pleasure and connection during intimate encounters, people may improve their emotional relationships and grow closer and more connected to their partners.

Touch and sensation are crucial elements of intimate relationships since they provide access to pleasure, desire, and emotional bonds. By learning about erogenous zones, mastering touch techniques, and overcoming emotional barriers to intimacy, people can create moments of extreme pleasure and connection in intimate experiences, strengthening their emotional ties and cultivating a sense of intimacy and connection with their partners. Through mutual knowledge, exploration, and conversation, couples may unlock the secrets of touch and sensation, creating deeply personal and soul-stirring moments of connection.

35

> *SET THE MOOD FOR A SENSUAL ENCOUNTER WITH THE HELP OF CANDLES, SOOTHING MUSIC, AND FRAGRANT AROMAS. IT IS POSSIBLE TO HEIGHTEN HER AROUSAL IN A GENTLE, AESTHETICALLY BEAUTIFUL*

CHAPTER 5

CREATING THE PERFECT ATMOSPHERE

Establishing the perfect atmosphere for intimacy requires skill—a deliberate balancing act between ambiance, emotional resonance, and sensory stimulation. Setting the scene is essential for couples who want to deepen their relationship and become more intimate because it allows them to create an atmosphere that promotes relaxation, excitement, and emotional connection. Every element plays a crucial role in defining the atmosphere and mood of intimate times, from taste, sound, and fragrance enhancers to lighting and music.

Creating the Ambience with Music and Lighting the Illumination Effect

Lighting is significant in setting the proper tone and atmosphere for interpersonal interactions. A cozy, intimate atmosphere may be created with gentle, low lighting, whereas harsh or brilliant lighting may seem cold and unwelcoming. The right lighting mix is essential for creating a stimulating and relaxing space. Candlelight is often regarded as the ideal choice for creating a romantic ambiance. The mellow, flickering glow of candles creates a warm, inviting atmosphere. They also form subtle shadows and add a sense of intimacy. Candles can transform any space into a sensual retreat, whether placed artfully on dressers and bedside tables or arranged in clusters across the room.

In addition to candles, gentle, indirect lighting may create a romantic atmosphere. Floor lamps with dimmer switches, wall sconces, and string lights can create a diffused soft glow, making the room seem cozy and inviting. Couples may also replace harsh overhead lighting with smoother, more ambient lighting to create a warm, welcoming, and intimate room.

The Function of Music

Music is another valuable tool for setting the mood and atmosphere of private discussions. The right music may heighten arousal, reinforce emotional bonding, and enhance the intimate experience. Music may evoke many emotions and sensations, from sensual and calming to energizing and vivid. This improves satisfaction and intimacy by producing a multimodal experience. When selecting music for private occasions, it's crucial to consider the atmosphere and feeling you want to create. While gentle, love ballads or jazz masterpieces can promote intimacy and a sense of connection, upbeat, rhythmic music can provide a lively and dynamic tone to the encounter. The most crucial step in creating a soundtrack to enrich the experience and strengthen your connection is choosing music you and your spouse can relate to.

Taste, Sound, and Scent as Enhancements

For thousands of years, people worldwide have understood that smells may arouse powerful emotions, memories, and senses. Certain scents are thought to be aphrodisiacs because they heighten perceptions of arousal. Couples may create a multisensory experience that satisfies all the senses and deepens their relationship by incorporating scent into personal interactions. One of the most popular fragrances to set a romantic tone is lavender. The well-known calming and relaxing properties of lavender can help reduce stress and anxiety while promoting calmness and tranquility. Other favored smells for intimacy include sandalwood, jasmine, and rose because of their sensual and aphrodisiac properties.

To create the desired aroma in the area, use room sprays, scented candles, or essential oil diffusers. Couples experimenting with several scents might find which ones appeal to them the most, creating a personalized perfume that deepens their relationship.

The Function of Sound
Sound is another valuable tool for increasing closeness and arousal. Delicate and lyrical or rhythmic and pulsating music may foster a sense of exhilaration and anticipation for intimate moments. Couples can experiment with other noises, such as white noise or sounds from nature, and music to create a calming and serene atmosphere. When selecting music for private times, it's crucial to consider the atmosphere and feeling you want to make. Soft, relaxing sounds can help with relaxation and stress reduction, whereas repeated and pulsating noises can stimulate arousal and excitement. Playing with varied

noises may help couples create a diverse experience that appeals to all senses and deepens their relationship.

Taste's Sensual Quality
Chocolate, strawberries, and whipped cream are famous for enhancing intimacy since they are rich, decadent meals. Enjoy them as a pair, tasting the aromas and sensations and using their hands and tongues to explore each other's bodies. Foods known to increase libido, such as oysters, figs, and dark chocolate, are trendy. These meals are said to stimulate the senses and increase sexual desire, which heightens sensations of arousal and pleasure. By including these meals in their special times together, couples may foster an atmosphere of luxury and indulgence that deepens their relationship and increases intimacy.

In conclusion, creating the perfect atmosphere for intimacy is essential to enhancing emotional bonds, increasing arousal, and creating a sense of intimacy. Every element plays a crucial role in defining the atmosphere and mood of intimate times, from taste, sound, and fragrance enhancers to lighting and music. By carefully monitoring and incorporating these sensory cues into their intimate exchanges, couples may create a multidimensional experience that satisfies all their senses and deepens their relationship. The goal is to create a comfortable, inviting space perfect for intimacy—a sensuous refuge where passion and love may blossom—whether quirky, lively, or soft and sweet.

CHAPTER 6

COMMUNICATION AND CONSENT: THE LANGUAGE OF DESIRE.

Desire is the silent symphony that plays deep inside our souls; it is a tune of yearning and passion that whispers secrets to those ready to listen. The dance of flames beneath our skin is the primal yearning that fuels the fire of connection and wakes our senses. Spoken in the language of desire, words become poetry, gestures become sonnets, and every stare promises unfathomable joys. Speaking the language of desire is like unlocking the passages hidden in the heart, venturing into the depths of the soul, and succumbing to the alluring pulse of attraction and arousal. It is to bring our partners into the holy sanctuary of our wants, to embrace vulnerability with open arms, and to expose the pure, unadulterated essence of our most intense needs.

In the language of desire, every touch is a statement of passion, every kiss is proof of need, and every word whispered invokes joy. It's the language of the body, the heart, and the soul—a symphony of emotions that transcends spoken language and speaks directly to our hidden primal impulses. Communicating in the language of desire is analogous to dancing to the rhythm of your drum; it's an alluring interchange of vitality and purpose that arouses your senses and accelerates your heartbeat. It entails letting go of self-control and surrendering to the seductive embrace of passion to fully experience the boundless pleasure that awaits us beyond the boundary.

Defining limits and getting consent from each other:
Setting boundaries and achieving mutual agreement is like weaving a sacred place where trust, respect, and understanding create a safe and powerful atmosphere in the complicated fabric of intimate relationships. Ensuring that each partner feels heard, valued, and respected for their shortcomings and desires entails carefully balancing respect and want.

Recognizing the Significance of Limitations:
Boundaries are clearly defined and safeguard one's physical and mental well; they are not immovable walls meant to create division. They serve as quiet reminders to accept and embrace our partners' needs and goals while upholding our own. They are the gentle prods of dignity and self-respect. Recognizing each partner's inherent worth and autonomy is critical to fostering an environment where both parties feel free to express their needs and wishes without worrying about rejection or reprisals. This is the meaning of comprehending the fundamentals of limits.

Developing a Culture of Respect and Communication
Mutual consent and proper boundaries in intimate relationships are contingent upon efficient communication. The key is establishing a space where both partners are at ease and motivated to communicate

their wants, fears, and boundaries. An atmosphere of honesty, understanding, and openness. It is listening intently to one another's desires and concerns and attempting to understand rather than criticizing or ignoring them. Couples may co-create a shared understanding of each other's limits and wants by discussing carefully and compassionately, strengthening their closeness and trust.

Accepting the Consent Dance
Rather than being a fixed condition, consent is a dynamic, ongoing process based on mutual respect and understanding. Consent must be actively sought after and given with enthusiasm to ensure everyone feels free to communicate their desires and boundaries honestly. It's about respecting each person's inherent autonomy and dignity and their right to choose whatever makes them feel comfortable and safe. Accepting the dance of consent is about creating a culture of respect and empowerment where all sides feel heard, understood, and respected for their needs and desires.

Building a Sanctuary of Trust and Empowerment:
In conclusion, obtaining both parties' agreement and establishing boundaries in intimate relationships is a beautiful way to demonstrate love and respect. It also involves ongoing communication, empowerment, and self-discovery. It's about building a relationship based on recognizing and respecting each person's inherent value and autonomy, which fosters reciprocal respect, trust, and understanding. By cultivating a culture of open communication, empathy, and consent, couples may co-

create a sanctuary of confidence and empowerment. In this sacred space, love, desire, and respect combine to develop a relationship built on mutual understanding, respect, and empowerment.

In this environment of empowerment and trust, couples find solace in the knowledge that their opinions are valued, their boundaries are upheld, and they are supported. It's a safe sanctuary where love may live unrestricted by fear or judgment and where being genuine and vulnerable are valued. Together, couples go into this sacred area, discovering and developing as they deftly and respectfully negotiate the depths of intimacy and need. They embrace the beauty of consent as the cornerstone of their relationship and understand that true intimacy can only exist in an environment of mutual respect and understanding.

As they dance the delicate dance of intimacy, couples find strength in each other's weaknesses, comfort in each other's struggles, and joy in each other's achievements. They recognize that limits are expressions of their profound esteem and love for one another rather than anything that stands in the way of intimacy or a deeper understanding. In this space of empowerment and trust, where their link is forged by consent, communication, and respect, couples discover what true intimacy means. It is a relationship that reaches far into the spirit and touches the essence of what it is to be loved and to be loved. It transcends the material world.

As they enjoy the warmth of this sacred place, couples find solace in knowing they are valued, acknowledged, and seen for who they are. In this place, where love reigns supreme and intimacy has no bounds, one can feel safe, empowered, and trusted.

45

> *THOROUGH AFTERCARE IS NECESSARY. IT ENTAILS CONSOLING AND CARING FOR EACH OTHER AFTER INTENSE ACTIVITY, ENSURING BOTH PARTIES FEEL SAFE AND APPRECIATED.*

CHAPTER 7

MINDFULNESS AND PRESENCE

In addition to being in style terms, mindfulness and presence are practical techniques that may fundamentally alter our relationships, occupations, and overall well-being, among other aspects of our lives. The core of mindfulness is being fully present and engaged in the here and now without judgment or attachment to the past or future. It involves being open and curiously aware of our thoughts, feelings, sensations, and surroundings to better understand ourselves and the world around us.

Understanding Mindfulness

At its core, mindfulness is about cultivating an awareness that allows us to focus entirely on the present moment. It means being curious and open to our thoughts, feelings, and experiences rather than reacting immediately or becoming caught in a vicious cycle of worry and ruminating. This mindfulness practice may help us become more focused, peaceful, and straightforward within, which will help us deal with life's challenges.

The Influence of Being There

Although awareness of the present moment and presence are intimately associated, presence is more than that. Being completely present means putting all of our attention and awareness into whatever we are doing or experiencing at that moment. When we are really present, we are not distracted by thoughts of the past or the future. Instead, we are entirely absorbed in the activity, whether completing an assignment, spending time with a close friend, or simply admiring a breathtaking sunset.

Building Presence and Mindfulness

Living a life of consciousness and presence takes effort, persistence, and patience. Various techniques and activities, including mindful eating, mindful activity, and mindfulness meditation, can help us develop these qualities. It's essential to figure out what works best for us and to incorporate it into our daily routines in a way that feels authentic and durable.

Meditation with mindfulness

Mindfulness meditation is one of the most widely utilized and well-liked forms of mindfulness training. It involves choosing a quiet spot to sit and focusing on our breath, thoughts, and body sensations with an open mind. Regular mindfulness meditation may help us train our thoughts to become more composed, focused, and present, making overcoming life's challenges more accessible and evident.

Move with Awareness

Mindful movement practices such as yoga, tai chi, and qigong can help cultivate present mindfulness and mindfulness. Throughout these exercises, we move our bodies slowly and deliberately, paying attention to our breath and our feelings. Integrating mindfulness with exercise may help us become more aware of our bodies and the link between our minds and bodies.

Conscientious Consumption
Mindful eating is another helpful method for cultivating presence and awareness. It involves paying attention to the flavors, textures, colors, and scents of our food and the bodily sensations we experience while we eat. By eating mindfully, we may improve our understanding of the nutrients that food provides and our relationship to our bodies' signals of hunger and fullness.

The Advantages of Being Present and Mindful
The numerous benefits of mindfulness and presence are well-established. Research indicates that mindfulness can enhance emotional regulation, increase mental acuity, reduce stress, anxiety, and depression, and enhance overall well-being. Similarly, cultivating presence may help us become better listeners and communicators in our personal and professional spheres.

Including Presence and Mindfulness in Everyday Life
Practicing mindfulness and being in the present moment can be challenging, especially in a society where distractions are shared and time passes swiftly. Nevertheless, we may cultivate these qualities in many areas of our lives with commitment and effort. Throughout the day, we have several chances to practice mindfulness and present. Some of these include taking a moment to appreciate the beauty of nature, pausing to notice our bodily sensations while walking, or just concentrating on our breath while standing in line.

To sum up, cultivating presence and mindfulness may significantly improve our lives. Developing a greater awareness of ourselves and our environment may help us feel more connected, at ease, and straightforward. As a result, we'll be able to live more authentically and thoroughly. There are several ways to cultivate these traits daily, including mindful exercise, mindful eating, and mindfulness meditation. We must figure out what works best for us and commit to practicing often because we know the benefits will be worthwhile.

Methods to Remain Present

Sustaining awareness and focus during romantic moments is essential to developing deep connection, intimacy, and mutual understanding between lovers. Using mindfulness techniques in romantic interactions helps couples get closer and enjoy more fulfilling experiences. It's simple to become mired in anxieties and diversions amid the daily chaos. When in a romantic relationship, you may stay present by using the following techniques:

1. Conscious Breathing:
Practicing mindful breathing lets you stay present in romantic situations quickly and effectively. Focusing on the sensations of your breath as it enters and leaves your body may calm your thoughts and establish a sense of groundedness in the present. Taking deep breaths may help you stay grounded and in the moment, whether you're enjoying a quiet moment together or having a private conversation.

2. Perceptual Awareness:

Using your senses is another helpful method for staying present in romantic settings. Permit yourself to lose yourself entirely in the sensory experience of being with your partner. Focus on soaking in all the sights, sounds, tastes, scents, and textures surrounding you. Whether enjoying a romantic meal, taking a stroll together, or snuggling on the sofa, paying attention to your senses may help you stay in the moment and connected to your partner.

3. Nonverbal Communication:

Nonverbal communication may help keep your partner alert and connected during romantic moments. Please take note of your partner's posture, facial expressions, and body language, and then give something back. Nonverbal cues that convey love, care, and understanding, such as a reassuring smile, a prolonged look, or a gentle touch, can foster intimacy and a tighter link.

4. Paying attention:

The capacity to actively listen is necessary to keep one's attention and involvement during romantic encounters. Instead of concentrating on your own ideas or strategizing your next move, give your partner your attention while listening to them with understanding and interest. Ask open-ended questions, affirm their feelings, and provide something in return for their responses to ensure that you understand them and develop a stronger relationship with them.

5. Letting Go of Your Expectations:
Letting go of expectations in romantic situations is critical to being present and open. Rather than being pulled into ideals of how you believe things should be or how you want things to be, accept and be grateful for the present. To be fully present and engaged in your relationship without worrying about the past or the future, embrace spontaneity, fun, and curiosity.

6. Gazing with the eyes:
Eye gazing is a helpful tactic for fostering intimacy and connection during sexual relations. Maintaining eye contact helps couples feel present and connected, allowing them to fully commit to each other in the moment. Eye gazing is a sexual technique in which partners maintain eye contact during intimate moments, enabling the intimacy and intensity of their gaze to deepen their connection and heighten their pleasure.

7. Sensual erotic awareness:
Bringing awareness and attention to sexuality is the practice of erotic mindfulness. By practicing presence and inquiry, couples may deepen their connection with one another and themselves, increasing their enjoyment and intimacy in the bedroom. To fully understand the richness and depth of the sexual experience, couples can engage in erotic awareness by concentrating on the feelings, thoughts, and sensations that surface during sex.

8. Conscientious Hands:

Mindful touch is a great way to be present and connected to your partner during romantic moments. Give your whole focus to the physical connection and touch sensations, whether you're holding hands, embracing, or engaging in other intimate activities with your spouse. You will deepen your connection and experience a greater sense of intimacy if you allow yourself to savor the warmth, sensitivity, and closeness of the present. Another helpful tactic for being in the present moment during sex is gratitude. By learning to value one another and the event as a whole, couples may increase their level of satisfaction and fortify their relationship. As an exercise in gratitude, partners should take a minute to thank each other for their bodies, each other's presence, and the pleasure they are enjoying during sex. Couples may thoroughly enjoy the occasion and the present by putting aside their concerns and other distractions with this modest act of appreciation.

9. Accepting Erotica Customs:

Sensual rituals may also help couples be present during sex by creating an environment of intention and attention during the session. Couples may slow down, connect, and enjoy the moment by engaging in these rituals, ranging from lighting candles to giving each other a sensual massage to relaxing music. By including sensuous rituals in their sexual practice, partners may build a higher degree of closeness, pleasure, and connection.

10. Letting Go of Expectations:
In the end, giving up expectations is necessary to be present during sexual activity. If a couple is focused on achieving a specific objective or performance criteria, it may cause tension and worry that interferes with their quality time together. By letting go of expectations and allowing the experience to unfold naturally, couples may fully embrace the pleasure and connection they're experiencing and completely unwind into the moment. This sensation of yielding will enable partners to be present, engaged, and connected during sex, which enhances their pleasure and fulfillment.

Accepting Conscious Sexual Presence
Lastly, it should be mentioned that sex healing involves being present and may improve closeness, satisfaction, and connection between partners. By being alert and aware of their surroundings, couples may create a more intimate, trustworthy, and enjoyable setting in the bedroom. By being present in the moment and engaging in mindfulness breathing, sensory awareness, and sensitive attention, couples may enhance their enjoyment and connection. By practicing mindfulness together, couples may strengthen and deepen their bond and experience greater intimacy, satisfaction, and pleasure in their sexual connection.

Conscious Touch and Relationship
With thoughtful touch and connection during sex, intimate relationships may be altered to reach new heights of delight, pleasure, and connection. Mindfulness plays a significant role in helping partners in intimate

relationships become acutely aware of their bodies, feelings, and experiences. As a result, they become closer and relish each embrace, contact, and caress. By approaching sex with awareness and presence, couples may transcend the limitations of the physical body and discover the boundless possibilities of their shared relationship. Deeper connection, trust, and satisfaction are fostered as a result.

Knowing About Mindful Sexual Interaction

Mindful Sex: What Is It?
Couples may completely participate in each moment of sexual contact with clarity, openness, and responsiveness by practicing mindfulness and presence throughout. We call this attentive sex. It involves being aware of the thoughts, feelings, and emotions that arise during sex and forging a close relationship with oneself and one's partner. Instead of aiming for a specific outcome or goal, the concept of mindful sex is to accept and be interested in the experience as it unfolds minute by minute.

Mindful Sexual Practices' Advantages
Mindful sex has several advantages for couples, both as a unit and as individuals. The practice of mindful sex may enhance every aspect of the sexual experience, from greater connection and communication to closer proximity and pleasure.

Increased Enjoyment:
By being careful and conscious of their bodies, couples may increase their emotions of arousal and pleasure, leading to a more satisfying and enjoyable sexual encounter.

Greater Bond:
Mindful sex improves the feeling of intimacy and connection between partners by fostering an atmosphere that is open to vulnerability, trust, and candid discourse. By approaching sex with presence and intention, couples may strengthen their emotional bond and gain a better understanding of each other's needs, boundaries, and desires.

Enhanced Interaction:
Mindful couples can better speak honestly and freely, clearly and empathetically, expressing their needs, wants, and boundaries. By mindfully and presence-based communicating while negotiating the complexities of physical intimacy, couples may improve their bond and enjoyment of each other's company. This practice cultivates compassion and grace.

Developing Intentional Touch and Bonding During Intercourse

Establishing a Hallowed Area
Creating a holy place for introspective sex is essential to building intimacy, security, and trust in the relationship. This space might be physical, such as a serene outdoor

setting or a cozy bedroom, or it can be emotional, created via the cultivation of openness, vulnerability, and respect for one another. By establishing a holy space for thoughtful sex, a couple may create an environment that is beneficial to deepening their relationship and enhancing their enjoyment.

Using the Senses

Engaging their senses during attentive sex is essential for couples to experience their relationships' richness and depth fully. Every feeling, from the warmth of breath to the smoothness of skin, is a gateway to a deeper awareness and connection. By exercising mindfulness and awareness of the sensations of touch, taste, smell, and sound, couples may gain a greater understanding of the complexity and beauty of their sexual connection.

Speaking with Presence

Communication is essential to mindful sex because it allows couples to express their needs, desires, and boundaries in a clear and caring manner. By talking with awareness and presence, couples better understand each other's preferences and create a place where both partners feel seen, heard, and valued. By being open and sincere with one another, couples may gracefully and sensitively navigate the difficulties that come with sexual intimacy. This will strengthen the relationship and increase the sense of mutual fulfillment.

The Conscious Sexual Practice

Conscious Breathing

Mindful breathing is a primary mindful sex method that helps partners connect with their bodies and senses, ground themselves in the present moment, and ground themselves together. By using mindfulness and breath-centered relaxation techniques, couples may ease tension and anxiety and make space for more connection.

Feeling Concentration

In the mindfulness practice of "sentient concentration," participants inspect each other's bodies with curious attention, focusing on touch, texture, and temperature perceptions. Engaging in sensate focus activities may help couples become more intimate and connected, appreciate life more, and see the complex beauty of their bodies on a deeper level.

Tantric Routines

Numerous mindfulness-based techniques for enhancing sex pleasure and fortifying a couple's relationship are offered by tantric practices. Tantra provides couples with a variety of efficient methods, from breath work and meditation to sacred rituals and energy work, to help them explore the depths of their sexual connection and expand their capacity for pleasure and closeness.

In summary, couples have a significant chance to strengthen their link, increase their enjoyment, and develop a presence in their sexual relationship through thoughtful touch and connection during sex. Couples may transcend the boundaries of the physical body and unlock the limitless possibilities of their shared connection by approaching sex with mindfulness and awareness. This will promote a more incredible feeling of closeness, trust, and mutual enjoyment. Couples can encounter the transforming power of presence via the practice of mindful sex, which enables them to connect more fully with one another, themselves, and the outside world.

TO HEIGHTEN THE SENSUAL MOOD AND EXCITE HER SENSES, USE YOUR VOICE TO MURMUR GENTLE NOTHINGS OR PASSIONATE WANTS.

CHAPTER 8

EXPLORING FANTASIES

A widespread and regular part of human sexuality is sexual fantasies. They are fantasies, wants, and situations that frequently materialize in the mind, offering a rich and intricate environment for sexual expression and satisfaction. The goal of this investigation is to learn more about the complex realm of sexual fantasies and their consequences for both individual and interpersonal development.

What Makes Sexual Fantasies Natural?

The variety of sexual fantasies is matched by the individuals who have them. They range from brief ideas to complex, well-developed situations. These fantasies may feature actual persons, made-up characters, or ideas. Numerous things, such as psychological makeup, personal experiences, and cultural background, might impact them.

Sexual Fantasies Types
1. Common Fantasies: These include scenarios like role-playing, romantic encounters, and experimenting with power relations (e.g., dominance and submission) that many people would find interesting.
2. Taboo Fantasies: These contain aspects often considered improper or prohibited by society. These fantasies can be a safe place to explore urges that one would not act on in real life despite social taboos.

3. Fantasies Concerning Novelty: These comprise situations involving novel or unexplored experiences, such as interacting with several partners, attempting novel sexual approaches, or exploring various environments.

The Emotional and Psychological Facets of Sexual Fantasies

Sexual fantasies have psychological and emotional components in addition to bodily desire. They can fulfill several psychological purposes:

1. Fantasies give a mental retreat into a world of pleasure and excitement, a way to escape from the stresses and mundaneness of everyday life.
2. Self-Discovery: People can explore many elements of their identities—aspects they would not express in real life—through their imaginations.
3. Emotional Connection: Fantasies can strengthen emotional ties between a person and their partner by creating new pathways for intimacy and understanding.

The Function of Society and Culture

Cultural and societal conventions greatly influence sexual imaginations. Popular culture, literature, and the media frequently influence the substance and appropriateness of specific fantasies. When a person's desires diverge from society's expectations, these forces can lead to conflict.

The Media's Effect

The way that relationships and sex are portrayed in films, television series, novels, and internet material may influence what society deems acceptable or attractive. This might increase curiosity and openness but can also put undue pressure and expectations on people.

Social Shame and Taboos

Society frequently stigmatizes particular imaginations as improper or abnormal. As a result, people may feel guilt or shame, which keeps them from embracing or exploring their impulses. Breaking through these taboos requires sophisticated knowledge and a welcoming atmosphere that promotes candid communication.

Sharing Dreams with Companions

Speaking with a partner about your sexual dreams is one of the most gratifying and challenging parts of exploring them. Intimacy, trust, and mutual happiness may all be improved in a relationship via effective communication.

Developing Transparency and Trust

1. Creating a Safe Space: It's essential to create a space where both partners feel comfortable sharing their dreams without fear of judgment. This calls for comfort, empathy, and attentive listening.

2. Gradual Disclosure: It's possible to share fantasies gradually. Establishing confidence and trust before pursuing more intense or personal dreams might be beneficial.

Recognizing Limitations and Consent

1. Mutual Respect: We must honor each other's limits. Not every fantasy has to come true, and it's critical to acknowledge and respect what each partner finds comfortable.
2. Effective Communication: Establishing and discussing limits helps to keep any exploration joyful and agreeable for both partners.
3. Exploring sexual fantasies has its advantages:
For both individuals and couples exploring sexual fantasies, it has several advantages. It can promote personal development, interpersonal dynamics, and sexual fulfillment.

Increasing Pleasure in Relationships
By adding diversity and excitement to one's sexual life, pursuing fantasies might increase one's level of sexual pleasure. It gives people the satisfaction and joy of realizing desires they may not otherwise be able to.

Enhancing Dynamics of Relationships
Emotional and sexual bonds can be strengthened by discussing and sharing fantasies with a partner. It fosters open communication, increases trust, and can result in novel and enjoyable experiences that improve the partnership.

Promoting Individual Development
Acknowledging and accepting one's desires might include a self-exploration journey. It enables people to face and

get over internalized shame or guilt, explore many facets of their sexuality, and comprehend their wants and desires on a deeper level.

Potential Difficulties and Myths

There are difficulties and misunderstandings around sexual fantasies, notwithstanding their advantages. Addressing these, we may foster a more positive and tolerant perception of fantasy inquiry.

False beliefs regarding fantasies
1. Fantasy vs. Reality: It's a frequent misperception that fantasies are an attempt to bring such situations to life. But imaginations frequently stay in the domain of the mind and don't always materialize into acts that take place in the actual world.
2. Shame and Judgment: People frequently dread being embarrassed or secretive about their dreams. It might be a relief to know that fantasies are a natural aspect of human sexuality.

Handling Variations in Dreams
Partners may have different imaginations or comfort levels in other settings. Resolving these issues takes mutual respect, discussion, and compromise.
1. Finding Common Ground: Exploring fantasies together might be facilitated by determining areas of comfort or common interests between the two partners.
2. Honoring Individual Dreams: Even if two people have different visions, it's still necessary to appreciate one

another's dreams. This regard fosters an atmosphere of trust and acceptance.

The Safe and Ethical Investigation of Fantasies

It's crucial to explore imagination morally and securely. This means being aware of hazards, ensuring that every exploration is consensual, and considering one's and partner's well-being.

Permission and Interaction

Consent is the foundation of any ethical investigation into fantasy. Ensuring both parties feel respected and protected requires open and continuous discussion about limits, comfort levels, and desires.

Safe Procedures

1. Establishing limits: Well-defined limits help avert pain or injury. It is essential to discuss and decide upon these boundaries in advance.

2. Using Safe Words: When necessary, safe words offer a clear and concise means of communicating the need to pause or slow down during a conversation.

Investigating one's sexual desires may be a very fulfilling and intimate experience. It provides a route to increased closeness, increased sexual gratification, and profound self-discovery. Through transparent, respectful, and communicative approaches to this research, individuals and couples can discover new aspects of their sexuality and fortify their bonds. A happier, more meaningful sexual life is possible when one navigates the obstacles and misconceptions involved in acknowledging and appreciating the range of sexual dreams.

EMPLOY ROLES TO EXPERIMENT WITH VARIOUS IMAGINATIONS AND DYNAMICS. TO GUARANTEE COMFORT AND CONSENT, BEFOREHAND DISCUSS LIMITS AND WISHES.

CHAPTER 9

INTRODUCING TOYS AND ROLE-PLAYING

Maintaining an exciting and happy sexual intimacy may significantly strengthen the tie between partners, which is why it is an essential component of romantic partnerships. Role-playing and the usage of sex toys are two good ways to add excitement and freshness to the bedroom. These components have the power to elevate regular sex into unique encounters that promote stronger emotional bonds and increased pleasure. This thorough manual offers a clear road map for couples wishing to expand the range of sexual activities they engage in by delving into the concepts of role play and the use of sex toys.

Recognizing Sexual Role Play in Relationships

Role play: What is it?
To explore novel dynamics and situations, partners in sexual interactions engage in role-play by adopting various personalities or personas. This might involve anything from straightforward situations, such as dressing up as strangers meeting for the first time, to more complex setups with elaborate costumes, props, and intricate plots.

The Advantages of Role play
1. Improves Communication: Role-playing encourages candid discussion of goals, limits, and dreams, which might enhance the relationship's general communication.
2. Enhances closeness: Couples can enhance their emotional and physical closeness by getting to know each other's unique personalities and dreams.
3. Boosts Fun and Creativity: Role play breaks up routines and injects a playful aspect into relationships by providing a platform for creative expression and enjoyment.
4. Safely Explores Fantasies: It offers a secure environment for couples to investigate and realize dreams that may not be practical or comfortable to carry out in the real world.

Typical Role-playing Situations
1. Stranger Encounter: Assuming to meet at a café or bar for the first time.
2. Authority Figures: Situations with instructors, managers, or law enforcement officials.
3. Playing patient and doctor in a medical fantasy game.
4. Historical or Fantasy Characters: Using historical, literary, or cinematic costumery.
5. Power Dynamics: This study examines submission and dominance using figures like master/servant or queen/subject.

Setting Up for the Role Play

Talking About Goals and Limitations
It's crucial to discuss limits, interests and wants honestly before engaging in role-play. Both partners must be at ease and enthusiastic about the possibilities being discussed.
1. Determine Interests: Talk about what kinds of situations each partner finds appealing and why.
2. Establish Boundaries: To ensure both parties feel comfortable and respected during role-play, clearly define what is and isn't appropriate.
3. Decide on Safe Words: If one partner feels uncomfortable during the role play, they should agree on a safe phrase or signal to halt it.

Getting Costumes and Props Ready
Costumes and props may bring realism and immersion to the role-playing experience. These might be anything from basic things like spectacles or ties to more ornate outfits and accessories.
1. Costumes: Depending on the situation, one can make their own at home using materials from specialized shops, internet merchants, or thrift stores.
2. Props: Without needing to spend a lot of money, basic props like notepads, stethoscopes, or phony ID badges may significantly enhance the experience.

Creating the Scene
Setting up the proper setting is essential for role play to be successful. The scene can be as straightforward or

complex as you'd like, but it should draw both partners into the conversation.

1. Pick the Ideal Location: Whether it's the living room, bedroom, or even a hotel room, pick a place that works for the role-playing situation.

2. Decorate as Necessary: Little details like moving furniture, lighting candles, or using particular items may change the environment and improve the experience.

3. Employ Lighting and Music: These elements assist in establishing the right ambiance and setting the mood.

Maintaining Your Persona

While maintaining character can improve the role-playing experience, it's equally critical to be adaptable and considerate of one another's comfort zones.

1. Embrace the Role: To improve the experience, give the character and situation your attention.

2. React Naturally: Pay attention to your partner's cues and movements while letting things unfold organically.

3. Retain Communication: Check in with your partner while being true to yourself to ensure they are comfortable and having fun.

Recap Following the Role Play

After the role-play, spend some time debriefing with your partner. Talk about what went well, what could have been done better, and any fresh perceptions or emotions that surfaced.

1. Give Feedback: Talk about the experience, emphasizing the parts you liked and the things you would change for the next time.

2. Thank your companion for their participation and willingness to try new things together.

3. Future Plans: If the experience was enjoyable for both of you, talk about role-playing exercises in the future and ways to improve your sex life in general.

Comprehending Sexual Toys

Devices or items intended to increase sexual pleasure are known as sex toys. They come in many forms, sizes, and purposes and can be used alone or with another person.

1. The most common kind of sex toy is a vibrator, which is intended to stimulate users through vibration. They are available in several shapes and sizes, such as wand massagers, rabbit vibrators, and bullet vibrators.

2. Dildos: Sexual toys that don't vibrate and can be used for penetration. They are made of silicone, glass, and metal and come in various sizes.

3. Prostate massagers, butt plugs, and anal beads are examples of anal toys that are intended only for anal play.

4. Couples' toys: These include remote-controlled toys and vibrating rings that may be used by both couples simultaneously.

5. Handcuffs, blindfolds, and other restraints are examples of bondage gear that may enhance the BDSM experience.

Advantages of Using Sexual Toys

1. Enhances Pleasure: Unlike manual techniques, sex toys may offer a variety of stimulation types and intensities that may not be possible with them alone.

2. Enhances Sexual Health: Using sex toys regularly may enhance sensitivity and blood flow in the genital area, which is good for your overall sexual health.

3. Improves Intimacy: Playing with sex toys together may strengthen the bond between lovers and promote open conversation and trust.

4. Explores New Sensations: By allowing people to experiment with new feelings and experiences, sex toys help to maintain an engaging and varied sexual connection.

Choosing the Correct Sexual Toys

Finding Your Preferences and Interests

Determine the kinds of stimulation or experiences that you and your partner are interested in before investing in sex toys.

1. Talk about your desires: Be honest with each other about the feelings and experiences you're drawn to.

2. Do some joint research to choose sex toys that both couples would find appealing by looking up various toy kinds and their features.

3. Start Small: Before advancing to more sophisticated sex toys, if you're new to the world of sex toys, begin with basic, approachable alternatives.

Taking Quality and Safety into Account

Prioritizing quality and safety while choosing sex toys is essential. Here are some crucial things to remember:

1. Material: Select toys made of safe materials for the human body, such as stainless steel, silicone, or glass.

Avoid toys made of porous materials, as they may house germs.

2. Reputable companies: Buy toys from stores and companies known for their dependability and safety.

3. Cleaning and Upkeep: Verify how simple it is to clean and maintain the item. Observe the cleaning and storing guidelines provided by the manufacturer.

Introducing Sexual Toys in the Relationship

1. Introducing the Concept: Treat the subject with interest and openness. Describe your interest in utilizing sex toys and how you believe they may improve your sex life.

2. Investigating Together: Look through the selection of sex toys and select items that both couples will find appealing. The process might be less scary and more fun with this cooperative approach.

3. Starting Slow: Start with less daunting toys and develop more complex alternatives as you gain comfort.

HER SENSES OF TASTE, SMELL, AND TOUCH MAY ALL BE ENHANCED AND MADE MORE THRILLING BY USING BLINDFOLDS OR EARPLUGS.

CHAPTER 10

MAKING USE OF SEXUAL TOYS

When used for solo play, sex toys can help people better understand their sexual preferences, explore their bodies, and have more enjoyable sex.

1. Experimenting: Spend time figuring out which toys and methods work best for you.

2. Self-Discovery: Make greater sense of your body's reactions by using sex toys as a tool for self-discovery.

3. Improving Masturbation: Add more diversity and enjoyment, including toys in your routine.

Couples Engage in Play

Using sex toys during partnered sexual activities can improve mutual enjoyment, closeness, and communication.

1. Combining Toys: To increase enjoyment for both parties, incorporate toys into foreplay and intercourse. This might involve playing with different toys to explore different feelings or utilizing vibrators during sexual activity.

2. Sharing Control: Certain toys, such as remote-controlled vibrators, allow one person to control the device to add surprise and excitement.

3. Combining methods: To get the most enjoyment out of your toys, utilize them in conjunction with other types of stimulation like oral sex or manual processes.

Improving Particular Tasks

Certain sexual activities, such as oral sex, anal play, or BDSM, can be improved with the use of sex toys.

1. Oral Sex: To further stimulate the genitalia or other erogenous zones during oral sex, vibrating devices can be employed.

2. Anal Play: Prostate massagers and butt plugs are examples of anal devices that can increase enjoyment during anal play. If you're new to anal play, always start with smaller devices and use lots of lubrication.

3. BDSM: You may enhance your sexual encounters with aspects of power exchange and sensation play by using bondage gear and other BDSM toys. Ensure that there are established safe phrases or signals and that all actions are agreed upon.

Combining Sex Toys and Role Play Scenarios

1. Medical Fantasy: A vibrating wand can be used as a "medical tool" during an examination in a doctor-patient scenario, improving the sensory experience and offering a lifelike touch.

2. Authority Figures: One partner may operate the toy using a remote-controlled vibrator, giving role plays between teachers and students or bosses and employees a surprising element of control.

3. Use toys with themes in addition to clothes and props to create historical or fantasy characters. For example, a role play with a medieval theme would have a "royal scepter" dildo, or a future scene might feature vibrators that seem very high-tech.

4. Power Dynamics: Handcuffs, blindfolds, and paddles are examples of bondage equipment that may improve the experience and create a more intense and immersive connection in situations involving dominance and submission.

Overcoming Fears and Insecurities

Introducing sex toys and role-playing can occasionally trigger worries or insecurities in one or both partners. The following are methods to deal with and get over these obstacles:
1. Have an honest and open discussion about any worries or insecurities. Assure one another that these activities aim to increase your enjoyment and connection.
2. Take It Slow: Add additional components slowly. Begin with basic role-playing games and toys and work up to more intricate or intensive experiences.
3. Positive Reinforcement: Give encouraging remarks and words of support. Regardless of the result, acknowledge the effort and willingness to try new things.

Resolving Myths
The incorporation of sex toys and role play into a relationship might be impeded by misconceptions. It is essential to address these misconceptions:

1. Role-playing Fallacies
- Not Just for the Kinky: Role play may be enjoyable and helpful for all couples, not just those with particular fetishes.

- Not About Reality: Role-playing is about discovery and fantasy, not a desire for real-life situations.

2. Myths About Sex Toys:
- Not a Replacement: Sex toys are instruments that increase enjoyment, not a substitute for a companion.
- Not Just for Individual Usage: A lot of sex toys are made especially for dual usage by partners.

Ensuring Playtime Safety
When role-playing, safety is crucial, mainly when dealing with situations involving power dynamics or physical confinement.
1. Defined Boundaries: Before initiating any role-playing exercise, clearly define the parameters and restrictions.
2. Safe Words: Decide on signals or safe words that may be used to halt or suspend an activity quickly.
3. Respect and Trust: Reciprocal respect and trust are crucial. Check-in with your companion frequently to ensure that both of you are having fun and are comfortable.

Use of Sex Toys Safely
For the sake of cleanliness and safety, sex toys must be used and maintained correctly.
1. Read the Instructions: Comply with the manufacturer's usage, maintenance, and storage guidelines.
2. Body-Safe Materials: Verify if toys are constructed from non-porous, body-safe materials such as medical-grade plastic, silicone, or stainless steel.
3. Cleaning: Thoroughly clean toys before and after each use with the proper cleaners. Certain toys don't need

particular cleaning agents, while others are waterproof and may be cleaned with soap and water.

4. Lubrication: Since silicone-based lubricants can harm silicone devices, use water-based lubricants with the majority of sex toys.

Establishing It as a Routine

You may maintain the excitement and fulfillment of your sexual life by including role play and sex toys in your routine.

1. Plan Your Playtime: Allocate designated periods for experimenting with toys and role-playing. This guarantees enough time for both couples to emotionally and physically prepare.

2. Although planned sessions are fantastic, feel free to add aspects on the spur of the moment.

3. Continuous Exploration: Never stop trying new situations to avoid monotony and preserve enthusiasm.

Putting Together a Collection

Build a collection of costumes and toys that both partners will love over time. This can offer a range of choices and keep the experiences engaging and novel.

1. Start Small: Depending on your interests and experiences, start with a few simple toys and costumes and progressively add more.

2. Quality Over Quantity: Make an investment in sturdy, safe, and high-quality toys and costumes.

3. Storage: Store them correctly to preserve the cleanliness and condition of toys and costumes. Think about utilizing a special box or cabinet.

Constant Communication

Effectively incorporating role play and sex toys into your relationship requires constant communication.

1. Frequent Check-ins: Communicate regularly about what is and isn't working and any new passions or dreams.

2. Feedback: Provide helpful criticism while being receptive to it. This helps to hone and enhance both parties' experiences.

3. Emotional Support: Provide comfort and emotional support. New sexual terrain may be dangerous; therefore, assistance from others is necessary when navigating it.

Thinking Back on Past Events

Give your shared experiences some thought. You may use this to determine what elements of the session you liked most and how to make it better in the future.

1. Post-Play Discussions: Talk about what you enjoyed, your difficulties, and what you would do better the next time after each session.

2. Celebrate Your Successes: Give credit to the hard work and inventiveness that went into making your successes.

3. Learn and Adapt: Modify your strategy by using reflection to gain new insights. Every encounter offers priceless insights into one another's boundaries and preferences.

In summary, you may significantly improve closeness, pleasure, and communication in your sexual relationship by using role play and sex toys. Through an open-minded, respectful, and communicative attitude to these activities, couples can discover new aspects of their sexuality and deepen their relationship. Recall that the objective is to provide happy and pleasant experiences for both parties, encouraging a more satisfying sexual relationship and a deeper level of connection. This guide offers a detailed road map for integrating role play and sex toys into your private life, regardless of whether you're new to these ideas or want to extend your current habits.

INCLUDE MASSAGE WHEN ENGAGING IN FOREPLAY. APPLY LOTIONS OR OILS TO HER WHOLE BODY WHILE BALANCING EXCITEMENT AND RELAXATION.

CHAPTER 11

THE ABILITY TO IMAGINE

The ability to conjure up mental pictures, events, and experiences outside our immediate world is a profound and fundamental feature of human cognition. Imagination has the power to change sexuality; it may enhance our sex and strengthen our bonds with one another on an emotional level. This essay examines the many facets of imagination in sexual relationships, emphasizing how it may improve arousal, fulfillment, and closeness without the need for role-playing or sex toys.

The Imagination's Fundamental Role in Sexuality
The mental activity of imagining situations, feelings, and sensations that improve sexual enjoyment and connection is known as imagination in sexuality. It goes beyond the physical parts of sex and gives people and couples a confidential, secure mental place to explore their innermost imaginations and wants.

Sexual Imagination's Nature
Sexual imagination involves the mental and emotional processes that produce colorful and captivating images in the mind. It is impacted by media, cultural narratives, and individual experiences and can be purposeful or impulsive.
1. Cognitive Imagery: Creating mental pictures of partners, situations, or sex-related actions.

2. Emotional Resonance: Feeling the feelings of arousal, love, and excitement connected to these pictures.
3. Personalization: Adapting dreams to suit specific needs and tastes to create a singularly fulfilling experience.

Using Imagination to Boost Intimacy

Imagination may significantly increase intimacy in sexual interactions by strengthening emotional ties and encouraging a sense of closeness and understanding between lovers.

Emotional Bonding
Couples may use their imaginations to explore and communicate their feelings in impossible ways with only words or physical acts.
1. Emotional Vulnerability: When couples engage in imaginative dreams together, they can provide a secure environment to communicate their most intimate wants and anxieties.
2. Empathy and Mutual Understanding: Imagination helps partners see each other's viewpoints and experiences, enhancing mutual understanding and promoting empathy.
3. Emotional Fulfillment: By creating loving and caring images in one's mind, couples might feel more treasured and appreciated.

Establishing Trust
Intimate relationships are based on trust, and imagination may be vital to fostering and preserving trust.

1. Shared Fantasies: By fostering a secure environment for candid dialogue and acceptance of one another, talking about and discussing sexual fantasies helps increase trust.
2. Honoring Boundaries: Honoring one another's creative limits and desires builds mutual respect and trust.
3. Consensual Exploration: Imagination creates a secure and trusting environment for couples to explore new facets of their sexuality in a consensual manner.

Increasing Arousal via Imagination
With countless opportunities for thrill and mental stimulation, imagination is a potent tool for increasing sexual desire.

Expectation and Want
By conjuring up vivid mental images that can heighten excitement and arousal both before and during sexual action, imagination feeds anticipation and desire.
1. Mental Foreplay: To raise arousal and anticipation, one might engage in mental foreplay by visualizing sexy situations and feelings.
2. Long-Distance closeness: By imagining future meetings and shared experiences, couples in long-distance relationships can use their imagination to sustain closeness and desire.
3. Sensory Enhancement: During sex, imagining certain sensory aspects like touch, taste, and smell can heighten arousal and physical feelings.

Examining Dreams

People can experience a broad range of wants and scenarios in a private and secure mental environment by using their imaginations to explore their sexual fantasies.

1. Variety and Novelty: Imagination keeps sexual practices from getting boring by offering countless variations and novelties.

2. Safe Exploration: People can safely explore desires that would be dangerous or impracticable to pursue in the real world by using their imaginations.

3. Personal Fulfillment: Customizing dreams to fit individual interests guarantees a unique, rewarding experience.

Overcoming Obstacles with Creativity

Additionally, by overcoming obstacles in their sexual lives, individuals and couples can improve their sexual happiness and well-being by using imagination.

Dealing with Sexual Reluctance

When it comes to overcoming sexual inhibitions and self-consciousness, imagination may be an effective technique that helps people feel more at ease and confident.

1. Mental Exercise: Creating sexual scenarios in one's mind can increase one's comfort level and self-assurance in one's sexual ability.

2. Reducing Anxiety: You can relax and feel less nervous when you visualize having enjoyable and good sex.

3. Self-Acceptance: Imagination can promote self-acceptance by enabling people to investigate and accept their aspirations without fear of criticism.

Improving Intercourse

Better sexual communication may be facilitated by using imagination to create a framework for talking about preferences, limits, and wants.

1. Descriptive Language: Partners may express their preferences and wishes more successfully using creative descriptions.

2. Imagination fosters creative expression, facilitating the discussion of complex or delicate subjects.

3. Mutual Exploration: Imaginative talks that explore the parties' wants may improve intimacy and understanding.

Imagination in Various Situations

The function of imagination in sexuality can change depending on the situation, such as when it comes to coupled sex, solo exploration, and cultural influences.

Individual Research

When it comes to solitary sexual exploration, imagination is essential since it offers a diverse and rich mental environment for self-gratification and exploration.

1. Personal Fantasies: People can develop and investigate personal fantasies that suit their interests and needs.

2. Self-Discovery: Through imaginative inquiry, one might become more aware of one's sexual identity and wants.

3. Emotional Connection: Imagination may help people feel more emotionally connected to themselves, which promotes acceptance and self-love.

Combined Sexual Activity

Imagination can improve the shared sexual experience in coupled sex, increasing closeness and satisfying both parties.

1. Shared Imagery: Partners should collaborate and imagine various situations to improve their arousal and sexual connection.

2. Emotional Bonding: Partners' emotional ties can be reinforced by envisioning tender and caring situations.

3. Improved Communication: Talking about and discussing creative fantasies can enhance understanding between partners and enhance sexual communication.

Cultural Affects

Cultural narratives and media can significantly influence our imaginations and desires around sexuality.

1. Media and Literature: Films, books, and other erotica offer a wealth of material for sexual imagination, generating new worlds and imaginations.

2. Cultural Norms: What is deemed desirable or acceptable may be shaped by cultural norms and taboos, which can affect the content and expression of sexual fantasies.

3. Social Dynamics: People can explore society's standards, and they might limit them by using their imagination to assist them in negotiating social dynamics and power systems.

Empirical Methods for Developing Creativity

Developing one's imagination can improve one's pleasure in relationships generally and during sex. These are some valuable tips for creating a rich and satisfying sexual fantasy.

Using the Media

Interacting with sensual literature, art, and media may stimulate one's sexual imagination by offering fresh concepts and possibilities to consider.

1. Reading erotic novels: Erotic fiction, with its rich and varied scenarios, may help you create new dreams and spark your imagination.
2. Watching Erotic Films: The vividness of creative situations can be enhanced by the visual and aural stimulus provided by erotic films and videos.
3. Investigating Art: Sensual art may stimulate creative inquiry and offer fresh viewpoints on attractiveness and longing.

Expression of the Creative

Imagination may be expanded via creative expression, facilitating the development of vivid and fulfilling mental situations.

1. Writing Fantasies: Putting your sexual fantasies in writing helps give them more substance and specificity, which increases their effect and pleasure.
2. Painting and drawing: Putting fantasies on paper might help people see them and gain fresh perspectives on their aspirations.

3. Storytelling: Telling and receiving sensual tales strengthen the creative bond and increase enjoyment.

Observation and visualization

Mindfulness and visualization practices can improve one's capacity to generate and maintain vivid creative situations.
1. Mindfulness Meditation: Mindfulness meditation can facilitate imaginative play by enhancing attention and relaxation.
2. Guided Visualization: You may develop intricate and engrossing sexual fantasies by engaging in guided visualization activities.
3. Sensory Focus: Emphasizing sensory elements like taste, smell, and touch may make imaginative scenarios more realistic and vivid.

Breaking Through Imagination Barriers

Some people can find it challenging to use their imagination in sexual situations, even if it has many advantages. These are some methods for getting through these obstacles.

Taking Care of Self-Consciousness

Being self-conscious might make it challenging to play imaginatively. It is essential to develop self-acceptance and confidence.
1. Positive Self-Talk: Using positive self-talk techniques can boost confidence and lessen feelings of self-consciousness.

2. Self-Compassion: Compassion helps lower inhibitions and promote self-acceptance.

3. Gradual Exploration: Introducing creative scenarios gradually can boost comfort and confidence.

Getting Past Cultural Taboos

Social norms and cultural taboos might limit one's capacity for sexual fantasy. It's crucial to question these conventions and embrace one's aspirations.

1. Educating Oneself: Acquiring knowledge about other cultural viewpoints on sexuality might offer fresh views and mitigate the impact of taboos.

2. Accepting Diversity: Acknowledging the range of sexual orientations among people helps promote tolerance and lessen bias.

3. Establishing Safe Spaces: Social restrictions can be lessened by providing secure and encouraging settings for sexual fantasy exploration.

Improving Interaction

Integrating imagination into sexual relationships requires effective communication about fantasies and wants.

1. Open Communication: To ensure mutual understanding and fulfillment, it is crucial to keep the lines of communication regarding sexual dreams and wants open and honest.

2. Active Listening: You may increase closeness and connection by attentively and sympathetically listening to your partner's dreams.

3. Respecting Boundaries: Establishing a secure and fulfilling creative environment requires that everyone respect one another's limits and boundaries.

In summary

A vital and potent component of human sexuality, imagination profoundly improves closeness, arousal, and fulfillment. Through accepting and

By developing their imagination, individuals and couples can discover new facets of their sexuality, strengthening their bonds with one another and improving their sex. There are countless opportunities for pleasure, fulfillment, and discovery in sex when one uses one's imagination, whether it be through shared fantasies, personal desires, or cultural influences.

PHYSICAL PLEASURE CAN BE ENHANCED BY EMOTIONAL CONNECTION. TAKE THE TIME TO STRENGTHEN YOUR EMOTIONAL CONNECTION BY HAVING IN-DEPTH TALKS AND MAKING LOVING GESTURES.

EMPLOY ROLES TO EXPERIMENT WITH VARIOUS IMAGINATIONS AND DYNAMICS. TO GUARANTEE COMFORT AND CONSENT, BEFOREHAND DISCUSS LIMITS AND WISHES.

CHAPTER 12

MAINTAINING INTIMACY IN RELATIONSHIPS

The essence of any love connection is passion. It stokes the first spark of attraction and maintains the relationship between lovers. Nonetheless, long-term passion maintenance calls for work, ingenuity, and commitment. This essay examines the complex topic of sustaining passion in partnerships, emphasizing the importance of foreplay at various relationship phases and the crucial areas of maintaining the spark.

Maintaining the Flame

A relationship's early flame frequently ignites easily, propelled by novelty and excitement. But sustaining this spark calls for deliberate action and conscious effort as time goes on. Here, we explore some methods for maintaining a burning desire in committed partnerships.

Comprehending the Spark

Before using any tactics, understanding what makes a relationship "spark" is crucial. The spark between couples results from a confluence of intellectual, physical, and emotional connections that arouse excitement and desire.

1. Emotional Connection: Maintaining desire requires a sense of closeness and connection fostered by deep emotional intimacy.

2. Physical attractiveness: The first spark and continual desire are primarily dependent on physical attractiveness and sexual chemistry.

3. Intellectual Stimulation: Having thought-provoking discussions and sharing similar interests keeps the relationship lively and fascinating.

Interaction and Emotional Closeness

Strong relationships are built on effective communication. It's more than simply talking; it's about actively hearing, comprehending, and reacting to your partner's wants and emotions.

1. Honest and Open Communication: Keep your lines of communication open and honest about your hopes, anxieties, and desires. Talk to your spouse about the things that thrill you and give you a sense of connection.

2. Active Listening: Engage in genuine hearing and comprehending your partner's viewpoint without passing judgment or interjecting.

3. Emotional Support: Offer dependable emotional support at trying times, demonstrating compassion and understanding.

Spending Quality Time Together

Spending quality time together strengthens the relationship between lovers. It allows them to create memories and experiences that fortify the bond.

1. Date evenings: Regular date evenings help keep your relationship fresh and exciting. Make plans for fun things that you both look forward to doing.

2. Common Interests: Take part in enjoyable interests or pastimes. This promotes a feeling of unity and purpose.
3. Travel and Adventure: Seeing new locations together may rekindle the enthusiasm and spirit of adventure that defined your relationship's early phases.

Physical Bonding
Having physical affection is essential to sustaining passion. It encompasses not just intimate sexual relations but also commonplace acts of kindness and affection.
1. Non-Sexual Touch: Small gestures such as kissing, embracing, and holding hands can strengthen emotional ties and closeness.
2. Physical Closeness: Consistent physical contact, such as holding hands or settling nearby, promotes safety and coziness.
3. Spontaneous Affection: To maintain the relationship, surprise your lover with unplanned displays of affection.

Maintaining the Novelty

The pursuit of novelty and excitement is necessary to maintain desire. Routine and boredom may be avoided by introducing novel experiences and maintaining a dynamic connection.
1. Surprise Dates: To keep your relationship fresh, schedule unexpected get-togethers or dates.
2. Learning Together: Acquire new abilities or take up new pastimes with your partner. This deepens the relationship while also offering new experiences.

3. Trying New Things: Keep an open mind and be willing to try new things, like a new dancing class, restaurant, or daring sport. New encounters have the power to rekindle the original flame.

Sustaining Uniqueness

Maintaining uniqueness is just as crucial for a healthy relationship as being together. It guarantees that each partner will develop further and infuse the partnership with new life.

1. Personal Interests: Support one another's pursuit of hobbies and interests. This encourages personal fulfillment and uniqueness.

2. Personal Space: Give each other's desire for solitude and personal space respect. This keeps things in balance and lessens the sensation of suffocating.

3. Self-Improvement: Make constant efforts to advance your development. A partner developing and growing in the relationship adds fresh vigor and enthusiasm.

4. Intercourse at Various Stages of a Relationship

A key element of sexual intimacy is foreplay, which has a varied function depending on the stage of a relationship. It includes preparing the mind and body for sexual action in addition to providing physical stimulation. An ability to modify foreplay in response to a relationship's evolving dynamics can assist in maintaining desire and improving sex.

The Function of Foreplay

In a sexual relationship, foreplay has several functions.
1. Increasing Arousal: Engaging in foreplay primes the body for sexual engagement and raises arousal levels.
2. Building Intimacy: It helps partners become more emotionally and physically intimate, strengthening their bond.
3. Raising Satisfaction: Good foreplay may raise libido and make the whole sexual encounter better.

Initiating Play in New Partnerships
Everything feels fresh and exciting when a relationship is just getting started. To create strong sexual chemistry and lay the groundwork for future closeness, foreplay is essential.
1. Boundary exploration: Utilize foreplay to delve into each other's preferences and boundaries. This promotes comprehension and trust.
2. Communication: Being open and honest about likes, dislikes, and desires is critical. This creates the foundation for a satisfying sexual partnership.
3. Playfulness: Make foreplay lively and daring. Try various approaches and pursuits to find out what interests both parties.
4. Emotional Connection: Put your energy into creating an emotional bond through close talks and similar experiences. Physical closeness is improved by emotional intimacy.

Long Term Relationship
Maintaining excitement and freshness in foreplay becomes harder as relationships go deeper. On the other hand, if deliberate effort is made, it may be a very fulfilling part of the relationship.
1. Routine vs. Novelty: Adding novelty helps keep foreplay lively even when familiarity might lead to routine. To keep people interested, mix novel experiences with regularity.
2. Deepening closeness: To increase emotional closeness, engage in foreplay. Intimate talks, massages, and eye contact are among the activities that promote connection.
3. Scheduled closeness: Making time for personal moments might help those with hectic schedules prioritize foreplay and sexual intimacy. Intimate plans may be just as thrilling as impromptu meetings.
4. Extended Foreplay: Make foreplay a leisurely and enjoyable affair by taking your time. Let each other's wants and needs come first; don't hurry.

Intimacy in Long Term Partnerships
Maintaining passion in long-term partnerships calls for ingenuity and work. Developing foreplay becomes essential to preserving closeness and sexual fulfillment.
1. Rekindling Romance: Rekindle romance with kind and affectionate acts. Show your sweetheart how much you care by surprising them with kind gestures.
2. Examining Fantasies: Talk about and investigate each other's sexual fantasies. This may heighten the climax and strengthen the sexual bond.

3. Physical and Emotional Support: Both emotional and physical support should be provided during foreplay. Recognize your partner's emotional condition and show them that you care by showing them empathy and affection.

4. Adapting to Changes: Adapt foreplay tactics to the way your body and your sexual demands evolve. Concentrate on what both couples find fulfilling and enjoyable.

Maintaining passion in a relationship is a dynamic, continuous process that calls for hard work, imagination, and commitment. Couples may make sure that their relationship stays lively and fascinating by communicating, spending quality time together, showing physical affection, being unique, and preserving originality. Furthermore, adjusting foreplay to fit various relationship phases might improve closeness and sexual satisfaction. To sustain sexual chemistry and strengthen emotional bonds, foreplay is essential whether a relationship is young, established, or long-term. Couples who use these tactics can maintain their passion and have happy, long-lasting relationships.

EMBRACE THE FUN ASPECT OF SEX AND DON'T BE SCARED TO LAUGH. LAUGHTER CAN HELP BOTH LOVERS UNWIND, WHICH MAKES THE ENCOUNTER LESS STRESSFUL AND MORE PLEASURABLE.

CHAPTER. 13

OVERCOMING DIFFICULTIES IN SEXUAL RELATIONSHIPS

Human connections are incomplete without sexual interactions, which also greatly enhance mental and physical health. It might be challenging to keep up a fulfilling and healthful sexual connection, though. To overcome these two typical obstacles, this post will explore how to manage desire disparities, stress, and weariness.

Handling Desire Discrepancies

In partnerships, differences in sexual desire are not uncommon and can lead to emotional detachment, dissatisfaction, and misunderstandings. Comprehending these distinctions and devising strategies to handle them may assist partners in preserving a satisfying intimate bond.

Recognizing Differences in Desire

1. Biological Factors: Individual differences exist in how drugs, health issues, and hormonal changes impact libido.
2. Psychological Factors: Emotional wellness, stress, and mental health problems all have a significant impact on sexual desire.
3. Relational Factors: Sexual desire is greatly influenced by relationship dynamics, which include emotional closeness, communication styles, and prior experiences.

4. Social and Cultural Factors: Cultural norms and societal expectations can shape individual views about sex and desire.

Techniques for Handling Desire Differences

1. Honest Communication

Navigating disparities in sexual desire requires effective communication. Discussing wants, preferences, and worries should be safe for partners without worrying about being judged.

- Honest Talks: Promote candid discussions around sexual frustrations and wants. Use "I" phrases to convey sentiments without blaming your spouse.

- Active Listening: Engage in active listening while demonstrating compassion and understanding for your partner's viewpoint.

- Frequent Check-ins: Arrange for frequent check-ins to talk about any shifts in desire and sexual satisfaction.

2. Comprehension and Feeling

Developing empathy and understanding might make it easier for couples to reconcile differences in desire.

- Educate Yourself: Gain knowledge of the variables that affect sexual desire, such as mood swings, stress levels outside of the body, and hormone changes.

- Empathize: Make an effort to comprehend your partner's viewpoint and feel sympathy for their circumstances. Refrain from assuming or passing judgment.

3. Flexibility and Compromise

It's crucial to find a compromise that satisfies both parties.

- Examine Alternatives: To preserve intimacy and closeness, think about non-sexual contact, snuggling, and kissing as alternatives to sexual intimacy.
- Be Adaptable: Be willing to try new things and modify your sexual schedule to suit the needs of both parties.
4. Get Expert Assistance
Occasionally, seeking expert advice is required to reconcile differences in desire.
Therapists and Counselors: A couple's counselor or sex therapist can help address underlying problems and facilitate fruitful dialogues.
- Medical Experts: Speak with a physician to rule out any illnesses that could be influencing your desire for sex.
5. Personal Self-Growth
Maintaining one's own physical and mental health might have a beneficial effect on one's desire for sex.
- Physical Health: Keep healthy by getting enough sleep, eating balanced food, and exercising frequently.
- Mental Health: Take care of mental health conditions like depression and anxiety as they might impact libido.
- Personal Fulfillment: Enjoy happy and fulfilling activities to elevate your mood and increase your desire.
6. Bringing Back the Romance
Differences in desire occasionally result from emotional distance. Sexual desire can be rekindled with a romantic rekindlement.
- Date evenings: To promote emotional closeness, schedule frequent date evenings.
- Surprise gestures: To express gratitude and affection, surprise each other with kind actions.

- Shared Experiences: To deepen your relationship, participate in novel and thrilling activities together.

Handling Exhaustion and Stress

In today's world, weariness and stress are prevalent and can have a significant influence on one's level of sexual desire and fulfillment. Taking care of these issues is essential to preserving a positive sexual connection.

Recognizing How Stress and Fatigue Affect Sexuality
1. Biological Effects: Stress releases the hormone cortisol, which can decrease libido. Fatigue diminishes physical vigor and interest in sexual activity.
2. Psychological Effects: Mental tiredness results from stress and weariness, which lowers one's ability to feel closeness and pleasure.
3. Relational Effects: Extended periods of weariness and stress can cause impatience, a breakdown in communication, and a loss of emotional closeness.

Techniques for Reducing Stress and Tiredness

1. Stress Reduction Methods
Effective stress management can raise sexual desire and general well-being.
- Mindfulness and Meditation: To lower stress and promote relaxation, practice mindfulness and meditation.
- Physical Activity: Engaging in regular exercise increases energy and relieves stress.
- Time Management: Develop better time management techniques to lighten workloads and make more time for romance and rest.

2. Enhancing the Quality of Sleep

Both general health and sexual health depend on getting enough sleep.

- Sleep Hygiene: Make sure your sleeping environment is pleasant, stick to a regular sleep schedule, and avoid using devices and caffeine just before bed.

- Treat Sleep Disorders: See a doctor if you have a sleep issue, such as insomnia or sleep apnea.

3. Making self-care a priority

Reducing stress and weariness requires self-care.

- Relaxation Techniques: Practice deep breathing, yoga, and massage as relaxation techniques.

- Hobbies and Interests: To unwind and rejuvenate, pursue your hobbies and interests.

- Social Support: Make sure you have a solid support system of friends and relatives.

4. Strengthening Emotional Bond

The negative impact of stress and exhaustion on sexual desire can be lessened by enhancing the emotional bond between lovers.

- Quality Time: To promote emotional connection, spend quality time together away from distractions.

- Emotional Support: During trying moments, extend understanding and emotional support.

- Shared Relaxation: Enjoy soothing pastimes like cooking, going on a stroll, or watching a movie as a couple.

5. Interaction and Comprehension

To assist each other more successfully, couples should be able to discuss stress and weariness openly.

- Address Difficulties: Be candid when discussing how weariness and stress affect a person's desire for sex.
- Offer help: To reduce stress, offer emotional and practical help.
- Have Patience: Show each other compassion and patience when difficult.

6. Expert Assistance

Getting expert assistance might help you better manage your stress and exhaustion.

- Therapists and Counselors: These professionals can offer techniques for reducing stress and enhancing mental health.
- Healthcare Providers: Seek guidance from healthcare professionals on managing stress, exhaustion, and any underlying medical conditions.

Combining Techniques for Extended Success

Sustaining consistency in motivation while managing tension and exhaustion requires constant work and dedication. Incorporating these techniques throughout daily life can result in long-term gains in sexual and relationship happiness.

Establishing a Helpful Environment

An atmosphere of support is necessary to cultivate closeness and reduce stress.

1. Positive Reinforcement: Congratulate and support one another on your attempts to improve intimacy and stress management.
2. Healthy Boundaries: Establish healthy boundaries to safeguard the time and resources needed for intimacy and self-care.

3. Shared Responsibilities: Lower stress, make more time for romance and relaxation and share domestic and family duties.

Frequent Self-Reflection and Modification

To keep up a good sexual connection, introspection and modification are essential regularly.
1. Self-Reflection: Consider your sexual fulfillment and general well-being regularly.
2. Joint Reflection: Arrange frequent check-ins to discuss how the relationship is going and what needs to be changed.
3. Adaptability: Be prepared to modify tactics when conditions alter and be receptive to fresh ideas.

Significant obstacles in sexual partnerships include navigating desire disparities and managing stress and weariness. Couples may overcome these obstacles and continue to have a long and gratifying sexual relationship, though, with open communication, understanding, empathy, and appropriate stress management skills. A supportive atmosphere that promotes intimacy lowers stress levels, and improves partners can create general well-being by emphasizing self-care, strengthening emotional connections, and getting professional help when needed. Couples may ensure that their sexual relationship is a source of happiness, connection, and mutual fulfillment by continuing to put in work and dedication.

CHAPTER 14

CONTINUOUS EXPLORATION IN SEXUAL RELATIONSHIPS

Sexuality is a dynamic and ever-evolving component of human existence, and it needs ongoing study and development to sustain closeness, pleasure, and relationship happiness. This article explores the value of constant inquiry, emphasizing the need to try out novel approaches and locate resources for lifelong learning.

Trying Out Novel Approaches
Intimacy may be rejuvenated, and the bond between couples is kept fascinating and new via sexual experimentation. It inspires couples to explore new interests, break out from habit, and have a more profound knowledge of one another's boundaries and wants.

The Value of Trial and Error
1. Improving Pleasure: Experimenting with different methods might bring up fresh feelings and experiences, which can improve your entire sex experience.
2. Increasing connection: Experimenting can promote a deeper emotional and physical connection as couples explore and learn together.
3. Preventing Monotony: Keeping a relationship lively and engaging requires regular experimenting to keep sexual rituals from getting boring.
4. Building Trust: Experimentation necessitates open communication and mutual trust, which fortifies the relationship.

Techniques for Conducting Experiments

1. Sharing Boundaries and Desires

For experimenting to be safe and fulfilling, there must be open communication about goals and boundaries.

- Expressing hobbies: Neither partner should be afraid to voice their curiosity or hobbies for fear of being judged.

- Establishing Boundaries: Before beginning any new activity, clearly state your boundaries and get everyone's approval.

- Active Listening: Engage in active listening to completely comprehend one another's wants and worries.

2. Initially, Make Minor Adjustments

Experiment with tiny, achievable adjustments to ease yourself into the process and gain confidence.

- New Positions: Experimenting with different sexual positions can offer novel experiences and variation.

- Different Locations: Adding some novelty and excitement to sexual activities might involve moving them to a new place.

- Adjusting Pacing: Try out various rhythms and speeds to see what seems the most enjoyable.

3. Investigating Sensory Interruption

Arousal and pleasure may be increased through sensory play by using many senses.

- Touch: Use feathers, silk, or other forms of touch to experiment with varied pressures and textures.

- Sight: To create a pleasing ambiance, include visual stimuli like lingerie, sexy films, or dimmed lights.

- Sound: To increase arousal, use music, sensual audio, or spoken conversation.

- Smell: Add aromas like candles or essential oils to create a calming and seductive atmosphere.
- Taste: To add a fun aspect to intercourse, try flavored lubricants or edible goodies.

4. Including fantasy

Fantasies may be a great place to experiment by letting partners try different roles and settings.
- Shared imaginations: To discover common ground and shared interests, talk about and discuss your imaginations.
- Role-playing: Introduce role-playing games to investigate various characters and interactions.
- Erotic Storytelling: Tell sensual tales to stimulate the mind and raise desire levels.

5. Making Use of Technology

There are several instruments available in modern technology that can improve sexual exploration.
- applications and Websites: Use applications and websites that walk couples through novel concepts and methods.
- Virtual Reality: Investigate immersive and interactive sexual material offered by virtual reality experiences.
- Remote-Control Toys: Try out these remote-control sex toys that your lover can operate even while they're separated.

6. Engaging in Mindfulness Practices

By lowering distractions and raising present-moment focus, mindfulness can improve sexual encounters.
- Sensate Focus: To improve your physical and emotional connection, engage in sensate focus activities.
- Mindful Breathing: Practice breathing to remain in the present moment and thoroughly enjoy your senses.

- Body Scan: To promote calm and heightened awareness of bodily sensations, practice body scan meditation.

Overcoming Obstacles in Research

1. Resolving Uncomfort

An inevitable aspect of experimenting is discomfort. Open communication about it can aid couples in navigating and overcoming it.

- Communicate Honesty: Be upfront and judgment-free when discussing discomfort or worries.
- Modify as Necessary: Be Prepared to modify or cease any uncomfortable actions.
- Provide reassurance: To allay worries and concerns, provide reassurance and support.

2. Managing Expectations

It is imperative to strike a balance between expectations and keep experimenting in a constructive and pleasurable way for both parties.

- Set Realistic Goals: Set reasonable goals for your experiments to prevent pressure or disappointment.
- Celebrate Little Wins: To boost confidence, acknowledge and appreciate little victories and fulfilling experiences.
- Have Patience: Recognize that not all experiments will yield results, and exercise patience throughout the procedure.

3. Preserving Consensus Between Parties

The basis for courteous and safe experimenting is mutual permission.

- Check-In Frequently: To guarantee ongoing consent and comfort, check in with each other frequently.

- Respect Boundaries: If someone withdraws their consent, all actions should cease immediately.
- Use Safe phrases: When conducting experiments, use safe phrases to express discomfort or the need to halt.

Resources for Lifelong Learning

To conduct an ongoing investigation, one must have access to trustworthy sources of fresh concepts, information, and direction. These are a few tools that couples may use to improve their understanding and experience of sex.

Web-Based Materials
1. Websites that Teach
Many websites provide instructional material on relationships, practices, and sexual wellness.
- Sexual Health Organizations: Information about sexual health and well-being may be found on websites such as the American Sexual Health Association and Planned Parenthood.
- Sex Educators: Pay attention to professionals who provide resources and expert counsel.
2. Workshops and Online Courses
Couples can take advantage of organized learning possibilities with online courses and seminars.
- Courses on Sexuality: Human sexuality and relationships are available on websites such as Coursera and Udemy.
- seminars: Hosted by sex therapists or educators, online seminars offer interactive learning opportunities and helpful advice.
3. Communities and Discussion Forums

Online communities and forums offer a space for exchanging experiences and talking about sexual issues.

- Reddit: Discussions on sexual difficulties and advice-seeking may be found in subreddits such as r/sex and r/sexover30.

- Sex-Positive groups: To meet others who have similar interests, join sex-positive groups on websites like FetLife.

Expert Advice

1. Sex counselors and therapists

Professional counselors and sex therapists can offer tailored advice and assistance.

- Individual treatment: To address specific sexual difficulties or concerns, seek out individual treatment.

- Couples treatment: Seek treatment for your relationship to enhance connection, communication, and sexual fulfillment.

2. Retreats and Workshops

Participate in retreats and programs aimed at improving your sexual interactions.

- Intimacy Workshops: Attend seminars covering methods for enhancing connection and intimacy.

- Sexual Retreats: Participate in retreats that provide in-depth instruction on sexual exploration together with professional advice.

Activities

It takes deliberate effort, mutual commitment, and purpose to include a continuous investigation into daily life. Here are some doable actions that may assist couples in preserving a fulfilling and exciting sexual relationship.

Establishing a Helpful Environment
1. Promoting Honest Communication
Talk freely and honestly with others about your sexual preferences, limits, and experiences.
- Schedule frequent Conversations: Set up frequent times to discuss fresh ideas or hobbies and sexual enjoyment.
- Non-Judgmental Attitude: Encourage an atmosphere where neither partner feels uncomfortable voicing their wants.
2. Making Time for Closeness
Set aside time regularly for closeness and sex exploration.
- Date Nights: Arrange frequent dates or special evenings when you can give each other your full attention without interruptions.
- Weekend Getaways: Occasionally go on mini-vacations or weekend getaways to explore new places and activities with your partner.
- personal Rituals: To preserve closeness and connection, create rituals like bedtime slumber parties or morning embraces.
- Scheduled Exploration: Assign designated periods for attempting novel methods or pursuits. This enables both parties to plan and prepare for exploration.

Accepting Inquisitiveness and Laughter
1. Inquisitiveness
In your sexual connection, foster curiosity and openness to new experiences.

- Exploring Together: View sexual exploration as a cooperative endeavor in which partners actively seek novel joys.
- Curiosity Exercises: To foster a more profound sense of understanding and connection, ask each other questions about your sexual preferences or desires.
2. levity
To maintain an enjoyable and thrilling sexual relationship, incorporate humor and fun into your interactions.
- fun Teasing: Increase anticipation and excitement, including flirting and fun teasing in your encounters.
- Sensual Games: Enjoy enjoyable activities that promote experimentation and discovery, or play sensual games.
- Laughter and pleasure: Savor the lighthearted parts of intimacy by embracing moments of laughter and joy throughout sexual encounters.

Developing an Attentive Mentality

1. Dedication to Acquiring Knowledge
Embrace a development mentality when it comes to sexual exploration, understanding that there is always more to learn and uncover.
- Learning Together: Seeking sexual exploration as a continuous process of mutual discovery is a great way to start a relationship.
Learning from Experience: Reflect on previous encounters and draw lessons from them, bringing fresh perspectives and understanding to subsequent interactions.
2. Requesting Opinions and Advice
Be willing to seek advice and criticism from one another and other resources, such as books, seminars, or experts.

- Feedback Conversations: After experimenting with new methods or exercises, have candid conversations about what went well and what needs improvement.
- Professional Advice: When faced with difficulties or inquiries, don't be afraid to see sex therapists, counselors, or educators.

Developing Closeness Outside of the Bedroom

1. Emotional Bonding
Recall that intimacy includes knowledge and emotional connection in addition to sensual pleasure.

Quality Time: When spending quality time together outside the bedroom, engage in activities that foster emotional closeness and connection.
- Meaningful Conversations: To deepen your emotional connection, have meaningful talks about your aspirations, worries, and wishes.
2. Non-Love Touch
To maintain physical bond and affection, include non-sexual contact in your regular encounters.
- Hugs and Kisses: Develop the practice of giving and receiving hugs, kisses, and cuddles throughout the day to show love and closeness.
- Massages and Caresses: As a token of affection and concern, give each other massages or soft touches.

Honoring Development and Advancement

1. Recognizing Success
Honor your accomplishments and advancements in sexual exploration, regardless of how minor they may appear.

- Reflection and thankfulness: Give some thought to your shared sexual experience and express your gratitude for the development and bonding you've shared.
- Celebration Rituals: Create customs or rituals to mark significant anniversaries and victories in your romantic partnership.

2. Accepting Your Imperfection

Accept that experimenting with sexuality is a journey with ups and downs, and learn to love the flaws encountered along the road.
- Self-Compassion: Show kindness and self-compassion to yourself and your spouse, particularly in complex or disappointing circumstances.
- Learning from Mistakes: Rather than seeing failures or mistakes as justification for self-criticism, view them as chances for development and learning.

Maintaining a healthy, joyful, and rewarding sexual relationship requires constant exploration. Couples may increase intimacy, strengthen connection, and maintain a dynamic and engaging sexual relationship by embracing lifelong learning tools, trying new approaches, and incorporating exploration into everyday activities. Together, with dedication, open communication, and a sense of adventure and playfulness, couples may embark on a self-discovery journey to improve their lives and relationships. Recall that sexual exploration is about development, connection, and shared experiences rather than perfection.

CHAPTER 15

EMBRACING THE JOURNEY OF INTIMACY

As we come to the end of our investigation into arousing desire and understanding the subtleties of foreplay in women, we must take a moment to consider the life-changing experience we have undertaken. We have explored the complex realm of female sexuality in this book, learning how foreplay may lead to deep closeness and pleasure. Now, as we say goodbye to these pages, let's embrace the knowledge gained and the experiences we had together, understanding that the path to intimacy is continuous and involves development, connection, and discovery.

Considering Our Journey Again

Our quest started with understanding the distinct nuances of female desire, realizing that it is complicated, multidimensional, and heavily impacted by emotional and physical elements. We discussed how important it is to comprehend personal preferences and wants, acknowledging that there isn't a single, universal strategy for achieving pleasure and arousal. Instead, we celebrated the individual paths every woman takes in her quest for satisfaction and accepted the variety of female sexuality.

Getting Good at Foreplay

The mastery of foreplay as a fundamental component of sexual enjoyment was at the center of our investigation. We explored the various ways that foreplay may heighten emotional connection, increase arousal, and spark desire. We discovered the power of anticipation and exploration in arousing desire and releasing pleasure, from sensuous touch to sexual conversation.

Handling the Details

Throughout our voyage, we carefully and sensitively handled the subtleties of female pleasure. We understood that communication, consent, and mutual respect are essential to creating a secure and encouraging atmosphere for exploration. We recognized that genuine intimacy is based on openness, acceptance, and trust, and we embraced the beauty of vulnerability and sincerity.

Accepting the Future

We know our path toward closeness is far from ending; therefore, as we wish these pages farewell, let's take forward the wisdom and insights we have learned. Let's keep exploring, growing, and learning—individually and collectively. Embracing the obstacles and achievements that lie ahead, we may see that they are all woven into the intricate fabric of the human experience.

Final Thoughts

Finally, let us remember that the path of intimacy is about relishing every moment along the route, not just getting to where you're going. Let's treasure the relationships we've built, the knowledge we've gained, and the affection we've experienced together. As we go on this incredible trip together, let's keep igniting desire in each other and ourselves.

EVERY NOW AND AGAIN, DURING FOREPLAY, LET HER LEAD. THIS GIVES HER THE FREEDOM TO DIRECT THE ENCOUNTER AND SHARE HER FAVORITE PARTS.

TOGETHER, READ SEXY NOVELS OR TALES. THIS CAN BE A GENTLE METHOD OF INTRODUCING NOVEL CONCEPTS AND MENTAL STIMULATION FOR BOTH PARTIES.